Resilient Youth: *Emotional Wellbeing in the Wake of the Covid-19 Global Pandemic*

Stories of Reflection and Resolve from the Trenches

Lisa La Bonté

Copyright© 2020 Lisa La Bonté

All rights reserved. No part of this publication may be reproduced, stored in a retrieval system, or transmitted in any form or by any means, without the permission of the copyright owner and Van Wagenen Publishing.

ISBN 10: 0-578-74730-3
ISBN 13: 978-0-578-75730-8

Book Design by Rabab AlHaddad

Van Wagenen Publishing
1101 Wilson Blvd
Arlington, VA 22209

Available from Amazon.com and other retail outlets

This book may also be ordered on our website:
www.SDGsChallenge.org/book-sdg3

Limit of Liability/Disclaimer of Warranty

The publisher, author and featured expert contributors make no representations or warranties with regard to the validity or effectiveness of the content of this book.

Please be advised that this book represents a practical and common sense approach to positive mental well being as shared through the lens of experience by individuals who are experts in their fields, predominantly management and innovation practitioners who have in some cases spent decades raising mentally strong and healthy children and/or working to instill emotional intelligence and enhance coping skills within young people worldwide.

For the most part, the author and contributors herein are NOT medical professionals or mental health experts - unless otherwise expressly referenced in/by their title and none of the content in this book should be taken as mental health or medical advice. The author and contributors make no warranty as to the accuracy or viability of the content and recognize that not all situations are the same in terms of feelings, moods, emotions, circumstances, outlooks, and mental health conditions.

The author and contributors do urge anyone struggling with emotional issues, whether mild or severe, to reach out to parents, family, friends, faith leaders, utilize a hotline in the back of this book, or seek private professional help if feelings become debilitating, overwhelming or dire. The organizations in the back of this book provide free professional counseling services, of which the author and contributors make no warranty expressly or implied. We wish all of our readers good mental health and wellbeing. Thank you.

Dedication

To the youth in this world facing an uncertain way forward and endeavoring to find their way each day amidst the upheaval, you are admired and loved.

To a world that has many ailments, Godspeed.

This book supports the UN Sustainable Development Goal (SDG) #3 Health and Wellbeing (for all by 2030).

It IS a Small World, Afterall

For many reading this book, nearly all shared a common bond before sharing a global pandemic.

On December 31, 2019 we were gathered across the globe, somewhere, alone or with a significant other, friends, family, and maybe strangers, as we celebrated the coming of a new year – the marvelously round number only added to the allure and optimism. 2020 represented a new decade – one with fresh resolutions, grand expectations and plans. And, literally, now, 2020 represents 'hindsight'. Looking back, 2020 started out well enough for many.

Change was Airborne

By the end of January, word – and an unknown, highly contagious virus was beginning to spread to all corners of the globe. Fast forward the past nine months (give or take) and Covid-19 has impacted –and inconvenienced – citizens worldwide – some obviously hit harder than others. Over 50 million globally have been infected, an estimated 1.2 million people have perished – and fortunately most have recovered over time.

And, through it all we questioned how and when our lives would return to some semblance of normal. For some of us our anxiety grew, we became stir-crazy and depression may have even set it. Still others managed change, learned to cope, and even rise to the challenge of the current circumstances.

And it turns out, introduced by this book's resident therapist Viva Goettinger, there's a psychological term as one rises from proverbial ashes, too.

According to Psychology Today magazine:

Posttraumatic Growth *"is the positive psychological change that some individuals experience after a life crisis or traumatic event. Posttraumatic growth doesn't deny deep distress, but rather posits that adversity can unintentionally yield changes in understanding oneself, others, and the world. Posttraumatic growth can, in fact, co-exist with posttraumatic stress disorder."*

The purpose of this book is to spur introspection and expanded self-awareness to enable healthy perspectives.

As you will soon see, this book maintains an overall theme of 'uplift' in an attempt to focus your attention away from the downer of Covid-19 while engaging your mind to nudge a pivot to the positives, to facilitate wellbeing or, if you prefer, to 'make lemonade.'

Table of Contributions

No News is Good News — 15
by Ayomide Ajakaiye, Nigeria

Note to Self — 18
by Olivia Zhi Hui Toh, Malaysia

Pandemic Poetry — 26
by Dylan Safai, USA

Decided Advantages of Down Time — 35
by Agusta Villalba, Ecuador

The Grace of God — 38
by Gracia Jeniefer, India

Life Flows On — 49
by Ryann Chalmers, USA

Close Calls — 54
by Sofia Bacanu, Romania

Making the Most of a Holding Pattern — 60
by Vivien Dimitrov, New Zealand

Life Changes — 64
by Fitia & Aro Robson, Madagasar

Finding the New Comfort Zone — 68
by Neo Mokhakala, Lesotho

Leap of Faith — 74
by Dhruv D'Souza, India

Keep Calm and Carry On — 80
by Katie Chu, Taiwan

Emotional Victory — 88
by Niharika D'Souza, India

The Sun Always Rises — 96
by Gladys Sophia, India

The Comeback — 102
by Moipone Selepe, Lesotho

Counting Blessings — 108
by Neha Varadharajan, India

Upward & Onward — 114
by Sydney Rico, USA

Tough Love & Guidance for a Good Life
Fatherly Widsom by Ahmad Jobain

Mind over Mood	118
Learn to Rely on Yourself	126
Hone your Personal Power & Fortify your Future	130
Failure is a Word not a Sentence	134
You're only as Dumb as You Believe	143
Selfish Sensibility	146
Ready, Aim, Shoot!	152
Celebrate Publicly, Complain Alone	156
Choose a Great Mentor	160
Neither a Servant nor a Stalker Be!	167
Read Rapaciously, Learn Lasciviously	170
Make a Plan & Accept the Consequences	174
Avoid Perfection	177
Make your Place & Be Seen and Heard	180
Minority Rules & Identity	184
Dare to Be Different	187
Life Isn't Always Fair	191
Your Body Speaks Volumes	194
What's your Hurry?!	198
Listen, Think, Speak	202
Humility is Overrated	207
Perspective & Perseverance, a Powerful Combo	211

Foreword

Embracing Posttraumatic Growth (PTG)

The stories in this book highlight how young people around the world are overcoming challenges during the pandemic. At a minimum, the 2020 pandemic has been very disruptive and in many cases it has caused a lot of suffering.

So how do we get to a more hopeful place in the face of such a difficult event? A concept called Posttraumatic Growth offers a way of thinking about this question.

Most people have heard of Posttraumatic Stress Disorder (PTSD), which some individuals experience after a traumatic event. It is less well-known, however, that another possible outcome of a difficult experience is Posttraumatic Growth (PTG). This is a concept that was described in the mid 1990s by psychologists Richard Tedeschi and Lawrence Calhoun.

PTG suggests that some people can learn and grow from a potentially traumatic experience in certain specific ways: to appreciate life more fully, to develop stronger relationships with others, to see new possibilities for their life, to find greater confidence in their own strength, and to grow in spiritual connection (https://ptgi.uncc.edu/what-is-ptg/).

What factors might help a person move toward posttraumatic growth? This is a question that is currently being researched, but we can make some informed guesses.

One of the most important elements is whether you have someone to talk to; a friend, family member, therapist, or other ally who can understand and accept what you are feeling. If you feel accompanied through a difficult time, you are much more likely to come out the other end with resilience and growth.

Another important factor that can lead to growth instead of breakdown is your mindset. Focusing on the good things that have resulted or may yet emerge from the pandemic as well as identifying your own strengths that have helped you manage and adapt are examples of a growth-oriented mindset.

Also important during a disruptive time like this is finding meaning in your experience. A life-changing event such as the pandemic invites reflection on such fundamental questions as:

- What is most important to me?
- What are the parts of my life that I see are valuable and need to be preserved, and are there any aspects that seem unnecessary now?
- Where do I want to focus my energy?
- What do I believe in, and have any of my beliefs changed?
- What motivates me to keep doing my best?

Youth (and adults alike) may want to consider these questions as they apply to their personal lives, or might feel called to consider them in the larger context of the world we live in. Many are likely aware of the various global challenges our world faces, and how interconnected so many of these problems are, including Covid-19.

This pandemic has been a hardship but also a wake-up call, showing us how quickly our lives can be drastically impacted when we are not actively working to address the imbalances our planet is facing. It can feel overwhelming to think about the scope of these challenges, yet more and more people are voicing their commitment to work for positive change.

Out of the difficulty of this pandemic, strength and resolve are emerging to care for our planet, the environment, the animals, and our own health and well-being. Appreciating what is most precious about life and believing in our ability to fight for what is most important; this is posttraumatic growth in action.

Viva Goettinger, Licensed Professional Counselor (LPC)

Preface

This book was created in response to a global pandemic, the likes the world's not seen since the Spanish flu of 1918. Likely no one on Earth recalls this level of havoc and panic over such a massive health crisis.

Many have experienced suffering related to financial or emotional health and a host of ancillary issues as we grow restless.

We've binge-watched HBO and Netflix, broke new video game high scores, Forged new Empires. We've blown up our social media, talked on the phone over chat or on zoom until we were tired of talking. We texted and whatsapp'd at all hours of the night (who's sleeping on a normal sleep schedule?). We ate mass quantities of yummy yet fattening comfort food to appease our emotions.

We were so bored, we actually read books! We caught up on the news online (we were dismayed by current events so we promptly stopped doing that!). Then, we ate some more. Surely we could use that diet app by now. We made so many tiktok videos and downloaded so many apps we ran out of memory and had to begrudgingly give our data to the cloud to free up space.

What else can we do? How many more video class sessions or business meetings, and virtual conferences can we endure? When will we be able to visit with our friends and families without having to wear a mask or social distance? How soon until we get dressed again and leave the sweatpants behind? When, if ever will life as we knew it return to 'normal'? How much longer until we have a vaccine?

We're coping the best we can, still, we want answers. Turns out, answers are elusive. More worrisome, the answers are constantly changing which further fuels uncertainty and restlessness.

There may not be many answers but so far we know that the physical, economic and mental health assault brought on by Covid-19 has affected much of the world population on varying levels – and in addition to the most vulnerable elderly, it's been especially tough on global youth – many of you reading this book.

That you are strong and capable of riding out this storm cannot be taken for granted. Surely we can all keep our cool a bit longer. Surely our days of climbing the walls are nearly over. But, what to do in the meantime to calm our minds, keep our spirits fed?

Let's embark on addressing and fortifying our emotional intelligence (EI). EI, if unfamiliar, relates to one's ability to be self-aware, understand, manage and control their emotions. A good level of EI enables coping skills and supports resiliency – and being resilient and rolling with the punches is what this book is all about. (Use the short unoffical EI test inside to learn your EQ!)

In an effort to address the issue of mental wellbeing, stories and circumstances straight from the source – teenagers from 6 continents – have been elicited and comprise the first half of this book.

The second half of this book consists of loving – yet, warning, bit of tough fatherly love, worldly advice to support well-adjusted youth provided by this book's resident Dad – a unique perspective and certainly fathers' perspectives are not heard nearly enough!

The ultimate purpose of this book is to provide a bit of uplift in a situation that's been a real downer and to help build the case that there is much positivity and constructive growth to be had by all, if only you take some time to consider the very bright light at the end of this very short tunnel.

Just when you thought you would run out of things to do to occupy your time and mind, tada!, this book arrives for you to 'do' (and a little reading, too).

Enjoy :)

Lisa La Bonte, M.S., M.B.A.

Interacting with this Book

Resilient Youth - Emotional Wellbeing in the Wake of the Covid-19 Global Pandemic attempts to provide some grains of sanity and inspiration along with humor and activities that reflect (and call for) creativity and positivity with the aim of providing some relief from common anxiety and frustration brought on by quarantines.

The stories by teen contributors have only been gently edited so as to keep the feeling and authenticity of their expressions, realizing that for many of them, English is a second (or third) language.

Ok! Time to take action and employ positive reflection, contemplation and distraction.

Gather your supplies: scissors, writing utensils, favorite coloring instruments, maybe some glue, and definitely some glitter! Channel the child within and start where you like - flip through the pages and start 'doing' to take your mind off the virus, the lockdowns, the disruption to daily life. If at least for a few moments here and there.

Pass the book around, if able to safely, and engage your friends, family, and co-workers in sections that are relevant for sharing or collaboration. As you can imagine, this pandemic will be one to remember and this book may serve as a memento to look back on, one day twenty years from now when you find it in a box of your old things in storage. It happens.

Upward and onward!

This book is dis-organized! on purpose, yet with purpose and there's a definite…

Method to the Madness, Sadness or Boredom*

~~Stop~~

Seize (C's!) Contentment and Conquer Quarantine

CREATE.................................... **draw or do** it

CONSIDER................................. **think** about it

COMMUNICATE .... **talk** about it

COLOR .... well, **color!** it

CRY..**release** it!

CELEBRATE .... **gratitude** in action!

Each C's activity type is interspersed throughout, in no particular order, and just enough jumbling of topics to keep you engaged (and healthily / hopefully, happily / distracted from this pandemic!).

You may see pages with a "Free Space" badge. These pages are either the backs (or fronts) of an activity for you to do that requires some "constructive" creativity… They can also be considered open spaces for you to jot down your feelings at any given moment in time.

* If your situation is serious, please find mental health resources at the end of this book, pages 214-215.

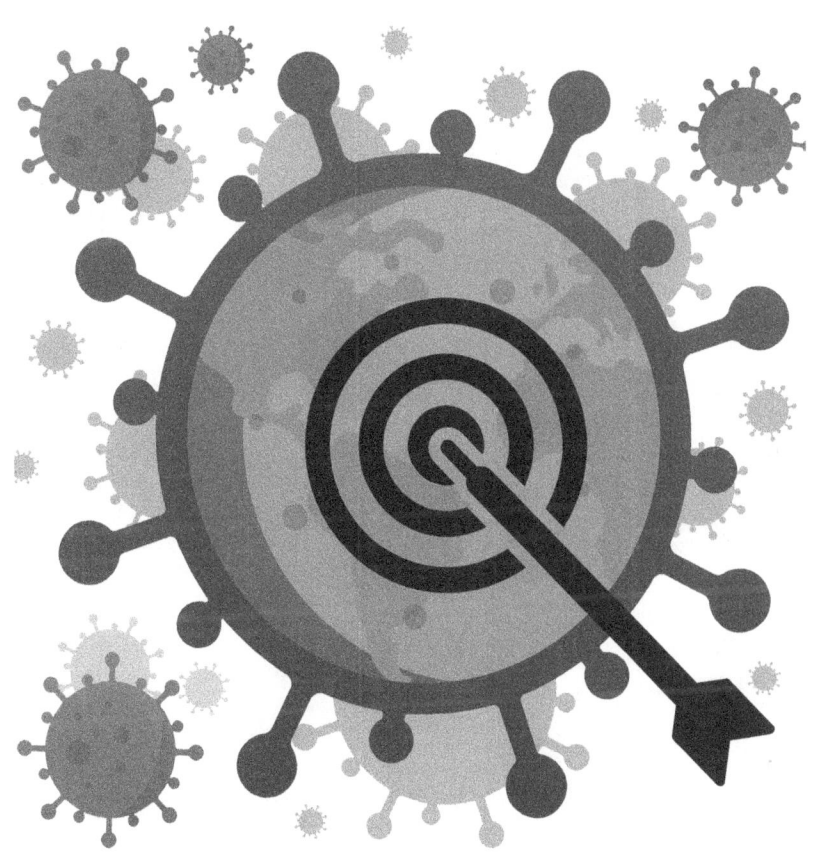

A SAD STATE of AFFAIRS

COVID-19 or Novel Coronavirus

According to the world renowned Mayo Clinic, "Coronaviruses are a family of viruses that can cause illnesses such as the common cold, severe acute respiratory syndrome (SARS) and Middle East respiratory syndrome (MERS)."

The Center for Disease Control in USA further states that in 2019, COVID-19, a new strain of coronavirus that had not been previously identified in humans caused an outbreak of respiratory illness first detected in Wuhan, Hubei province, China.

The virus is now known to manifest as severe acute respiratory syndrome and is called coronavirus disease 2019 (COVID-19).

Since December 2019, over 50 million cases have been identified worldwide resulting in over 1 million deaths.

In March 2020, the World Health Organization (WHO) declared the COVID-19 outbreak a pandemic.

Symptoms include:
- Shortness of breath
- Dry cough
- Body aches
- Fever
- Multiple and various flu-like symptoms

Those most affected include:

→ **Black population**

→ **Persons with co-morbidities (multiple existing diseases, esp. diabetes, obesity, cancer, hyper-tension) and compromised immune systems**

→ **Elderly persons with delicate or weak immune systems & Seniors**

Remain positive. If you leave home wear a mask, wash your hands frequently or use hand sanitizer and try not to touch your face! Practice social distancing and avoid large crowds.

Covid-19 Alert!

Need to contact your nation's Center for Disease Control or National Health Office?

> BING it!

Want up to date Covid information and statistics?

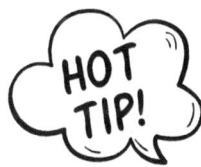

Don't google it, bing it! www.bing.com

When you use Microsoft's search engine, Bing, you GET REWARDS!

Earn Starbucks, Target, Amazon, Pizza Hut gift cards just by surfing the web like you do every day!!

Or, if you don't want gift cards, you can donate to a selection of charities!

And, Bing shares a new INSPIRING high-res photo every day :)

Get Up And Get Dressed!

Super Sites* to Help Make Positive Sense of Life!

LIFEHACK - as the name implies, all kinds of awesome tips and tools to hack a better life!

www.lifehack.org

"Be Kind to Your Mind" A free service if you're a student or unemployed, this site is EXCELLENT for mental health and wellbeing.

www.headspace.com

Check your IQ to see how you compare to Einstein!

www.test-iq.org

Mental workouts for a fit brain!

www.themindgym.com

Learn your **Myers Briggs Personality Type**!

https://cutt.ly/NgEBGe3

These are our faves –We'd love to learn about more, so email us yours! SDG3@SDGschallenge.org

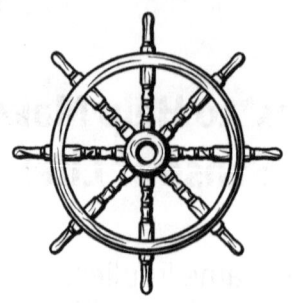

"I am the captain of my soul."
Nelson Mandela

and while you're at it, you can be the Prime Minister of your destiny.

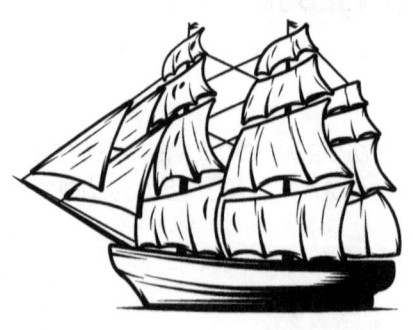

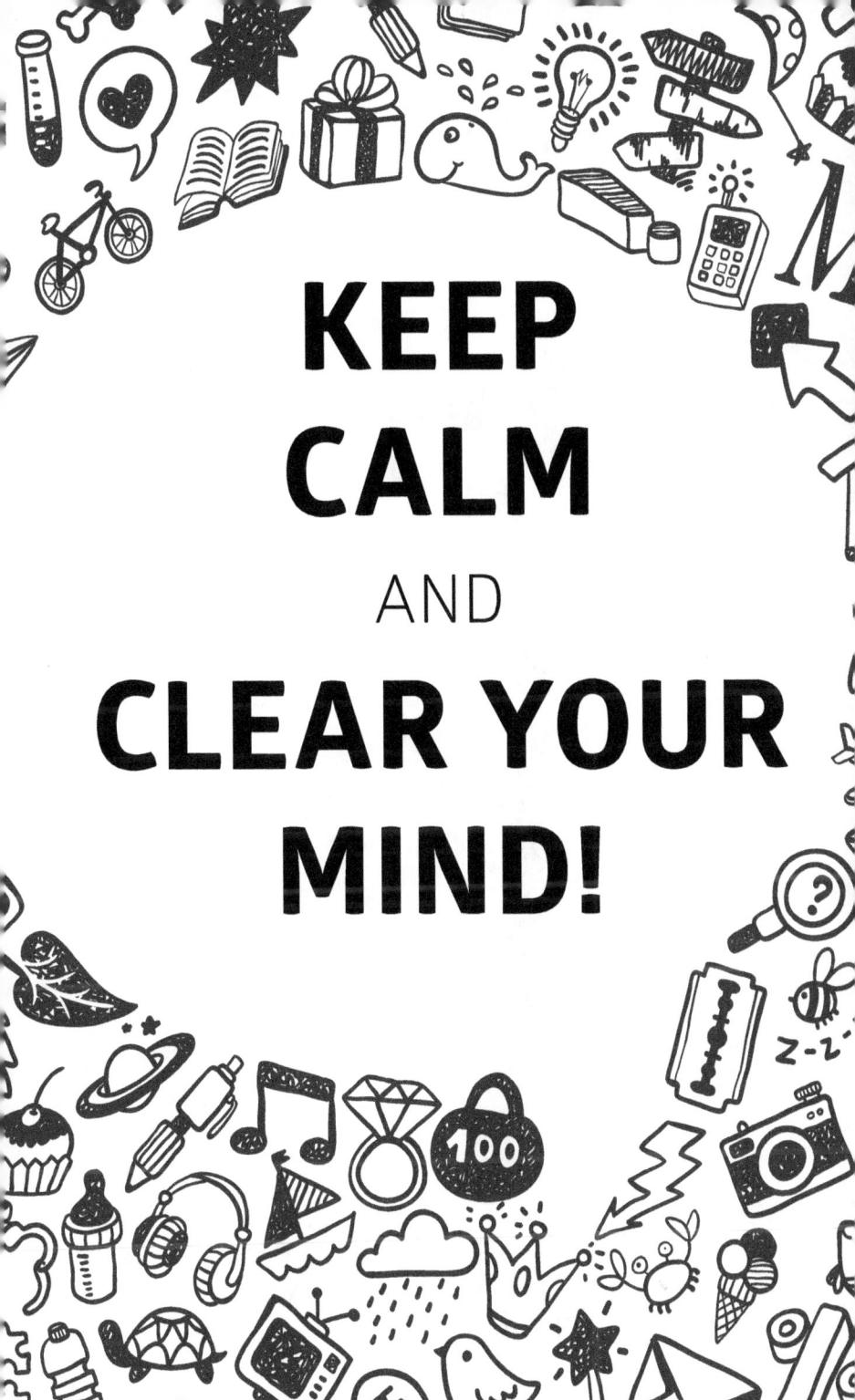

LIQUID LIFE

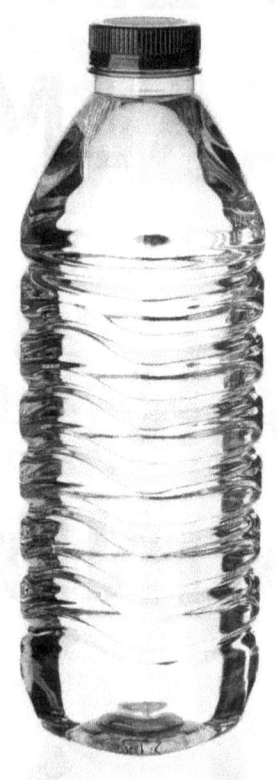

Did you know? Dehydration can cause headaches, poor digestive function, and... a really bad mood? Water keeps you human - and alive. Cheers!

List your

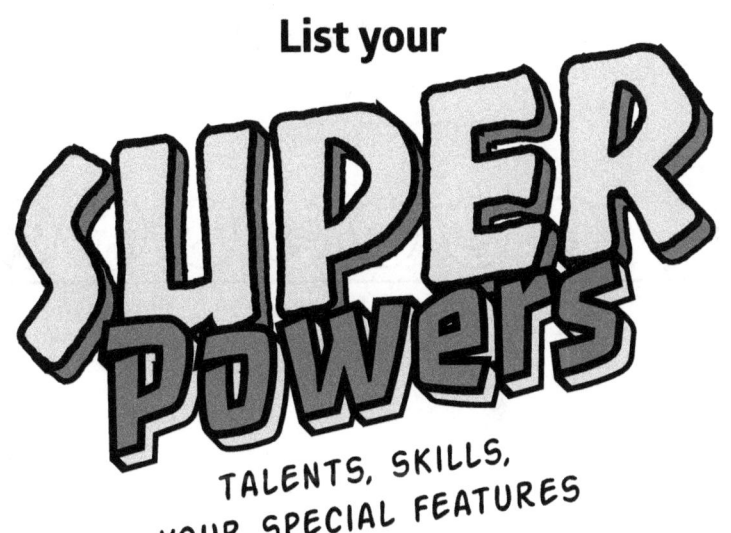

SUPER Powers
TALENTS, SKILLS, YOUR SPECIAL FEATURES

___

___

___

___

___

___

___

Mood tracker
2 weeks, try this fill in

Date	😄	🙂	😐	😳	🙁	😢	😠

If after 2 weeks you find mostly right side, please reach out to BFF, family, clergy, hotline, or others who can help.

The ills of Social Media

How Social Media Boosts Your Stress

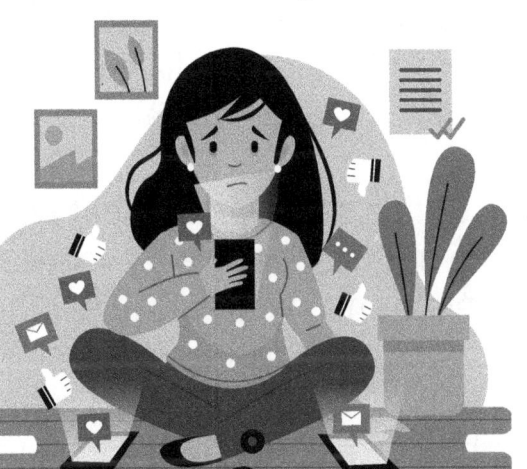

Find something to LAUGH at

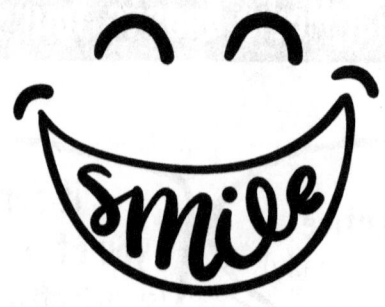

If you're online, look for a humorous video, watch your favorite comedian, comedy show or movie.

If you're offline, recall a time that was funny and laugh out loud or hold a zoom 'laugh in' with friends and see who can tell the best jokes or stories and wins the most laughs.

Laughter is a proven mood booster -- and aids physical health, too!

And, actual research shows that if you are down or feeling sad, forcing yourself to SMILE will start the positive mood endorphins in your brain!

No News is Good News

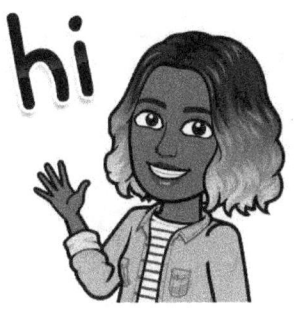

Through my several months of quarantine, listening to the news of US became a stream of despair, reminding me that society was not as perfect as it seems.

"Total US cases, worst in the world, surpass 5 million."

"The death of George Floyd, sparks massive global protests in America."

"Across the world the worst economic recessions in 3 generations."

These consistent jabs remind me that what I'm going through is not only out of the ordinary, but unfavorable. That things can get worse, when they already seemed bad, and that as a teen I'm trapped between the confines of my home, trapped behind its familiar walls, almost helpless to change it. It was like staring through a mirror and seeing nothing but scabs and wounds in the reflection. Unprecedented and the word normal almost had bitter taste in my mouth.

But eventually, as the months began to pass by, I learned to appreciate mirrors. My story didn't end with my first reflection. Multiple reflections tell the unique story of me. Mirrors can be reminders of our imperfections, but also motivations for our growth. The world doesn't end with this pandemic, not unless we let it. This virus can feel overwhelming, but it's important to recognize flaws so that you can improve. So that we all can improve. The world is filled with many scabs and wounds, but we must all band together to end these afflictions. So, that we can look at our newfound scars with pride because together we overcame them.

Ayomide Ajakaiye, 14, Nigeria

Grab your Blankie & some crayons, it's COLORING TIME!

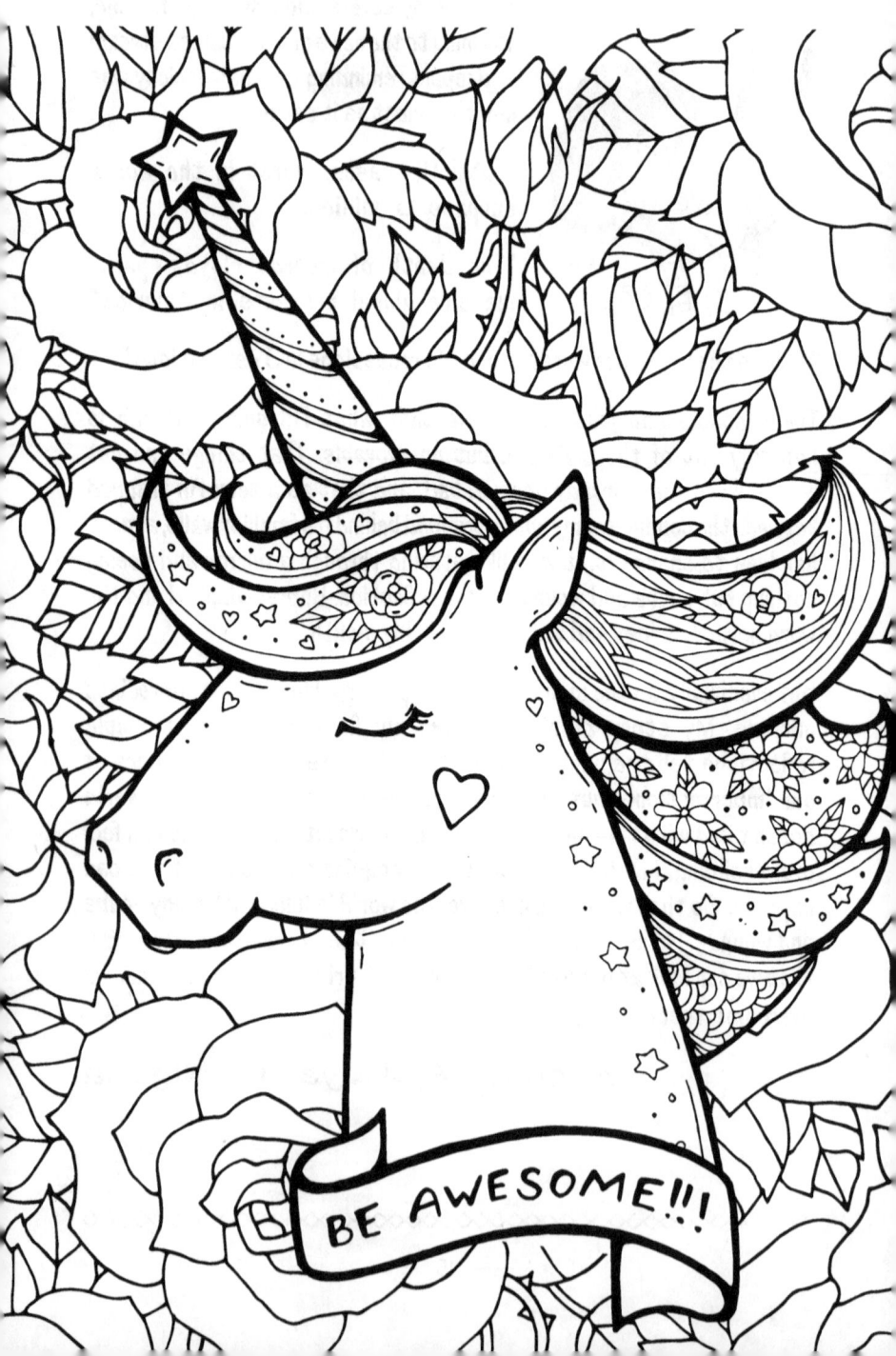

"Well done is better than well said."

Benjamin Franklin

So.... DO SOMETHING!

You have time now so perhaps...

Consider your future & MAKE SOME PLANS of things you want and aim to do!

Then, START DOING!

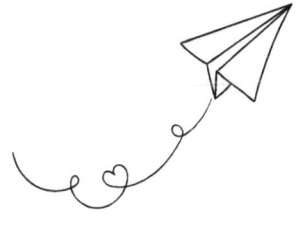

Note to Self

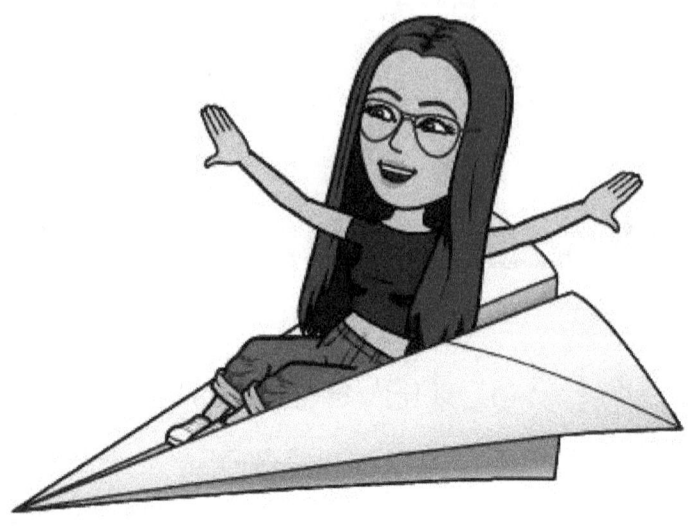

School, homework, eat, sleep, repeat. School, homework, eat, sleep, repeat. School, homework, eat, sleep, re—

The lockdown was an instant pause to my monotonous routines. Being used to rushing from one place to another, entertaining piles of work after work, the lockdown was a long-awaited hiatus - except some things resumed online.

I was apprehensive about the challenges virtual substitutes would bring. The fatigue from being stuck at home talking to screens all day, highly anticipated plans being canceled and sayings of a cursed 2020 seemed miserable at first.

However, gradually, I began to realize that things might not be that miserable after all. Just like the Law of Attraction, it all depends on which perspective our minds take on. Shift your vision to the bright side. I realized that everything happens for a reason and that beauty exists even when things seem gloomy.

The coming of the pandemic taught me to appreciate the bonds around me, no matter friends or family.

By witnessing how uncertain life can be, it taught me to cherish every moment I own; to never let fear hold me back, and take every opportunity I have to do things I want to accomplish.

It amazingly proved to us how we are all connected - a single device enabled us, of all global whereabouts, to support each other and stand united in our voices.

The lockdown was a period of self-reflection - a break for our souls. It shaped more mature worldviews and served as a time for us to truly discover things about ourselves. For me, I bonded closer with my loved ones, discovered new passions, and set new goals for myself - things I would never trade for anything in the world.

Dear You,

If you can't go outside, go inside.

Lots of love,
Olivia

Olivia Zhi Hui Toh, 15, Malaysia

◇◇◇

Let's get
O R G A N I Z E D

- Buy some new containers that are the same size and stackable to store all kinds of 'stuff' you can't live without

- Buy/use folders for loose papers

- Consider a new bookshelf or cabinet. Check Craigslist.org or similar online ad board for a free one or try Goodwill, Salvation Army or a local charity that sell old furniture - cheap! Do good at same time!

- Get stuff off your table tops, off the floor, off the bed! Go through your closet and weed out the old things you no longer wear (or... no longer fit you and won't again soon)

- Go through your...

PROMISE! You'll feel so much better once your space is in order and ORGANIZED!

Name 10 things that give you a feeling of Bliss

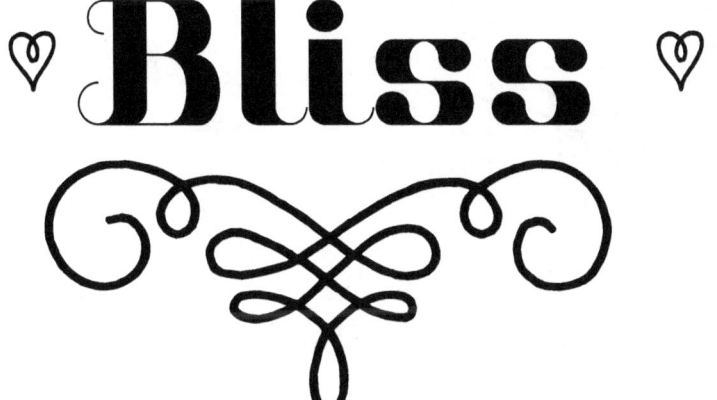

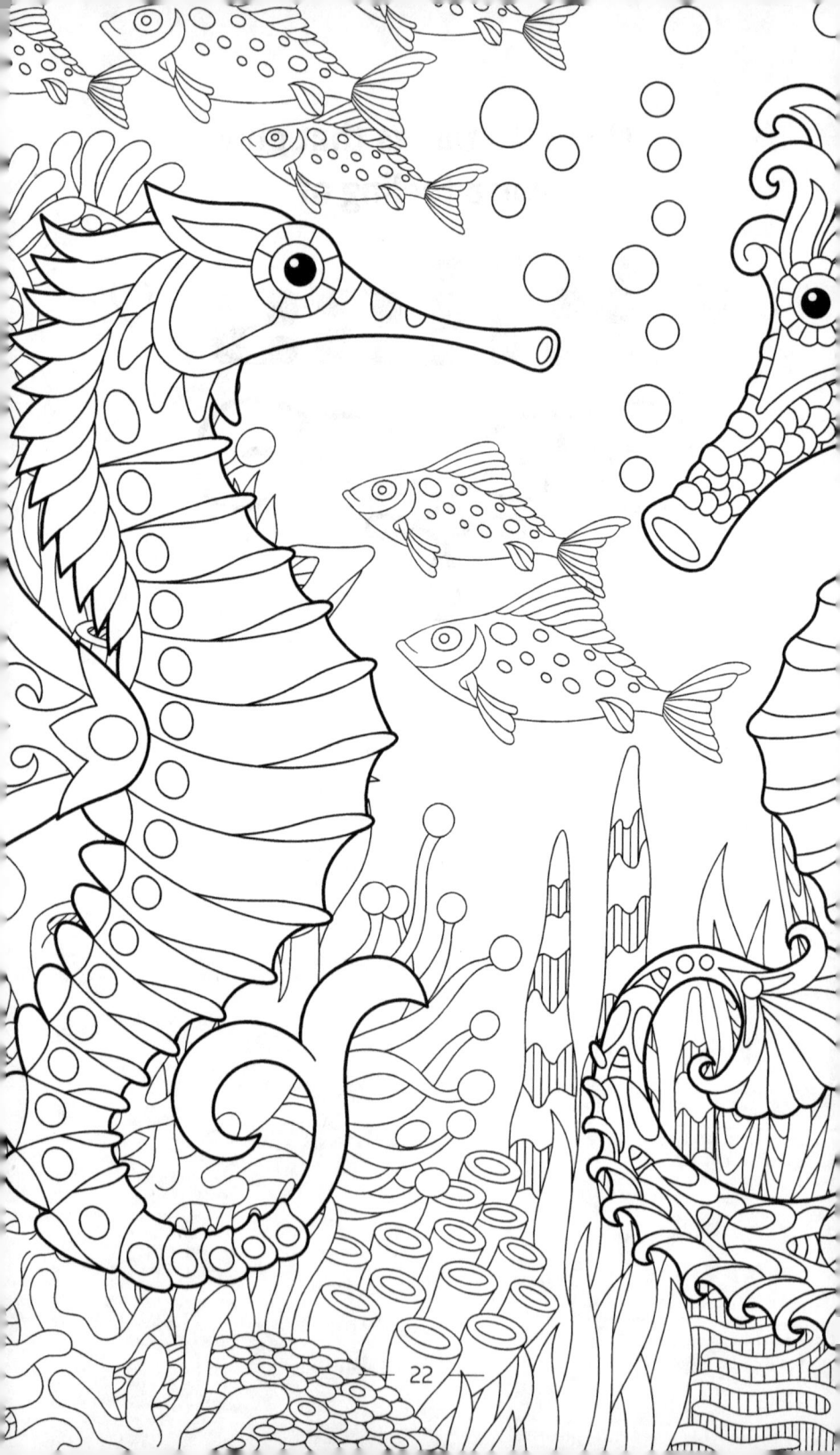

Stress Destruction

Take your frustration, aggression, irritation... out on this PAGE.

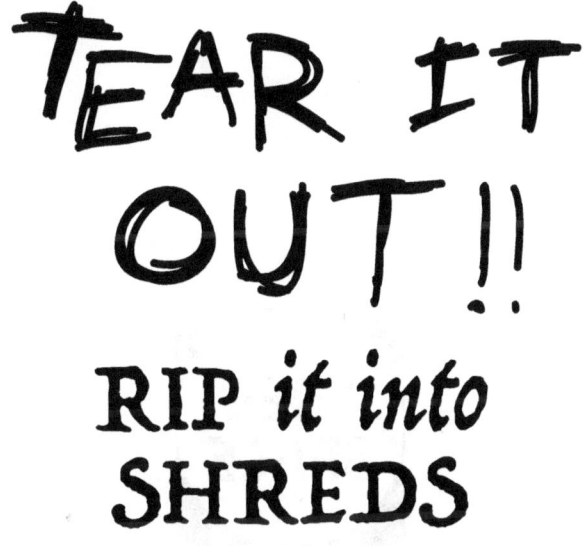

Make a loud, diabolical laugh like you see in the horror movies.

How many pieces can you rip it into? Record so far is 115. Certainly you can do better?

P.S. Put litter in its place.

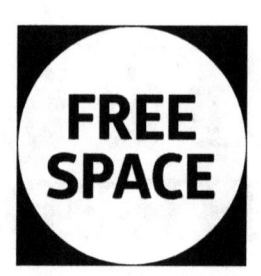

Having a difficult time?

Need new, non-judgey friends?

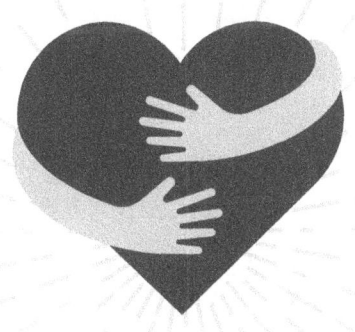

Reach out to us
(Use a confidential alias if you want!)

by email: SDG3@SDGschallenge.org
or
WhatsApp: +1 240 281 0307

Mention your
gender / age / timezone

♥ *we will connect you* ♥

Pandemic Poetry

Quarantine is a staircase with no end.
The days travel on, and continue to blend.
However, hope is in sight,
if we choose to look through the right light.

Some things that take up my day,
are getting up to go out and play.
Although school starts in the fall,
my only worry is dribbling my basketball.

Although covid cases have continued to grow,
I have learned how to soften its blow.
My advice for all to get through this time,
is to continue to think bright and shine.

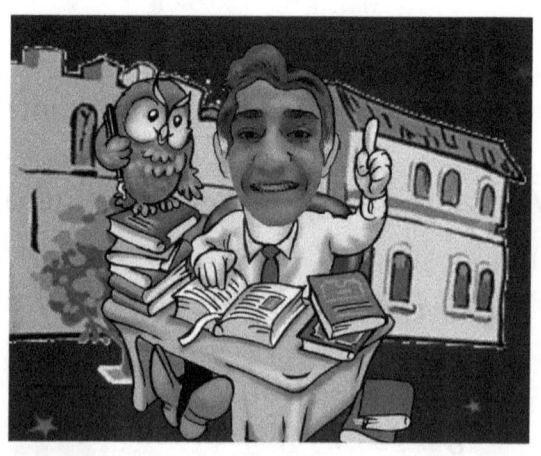

Dylan Safai, 16, USA (Persian American)

Add More ☼ to Your Life!

Sunshine is used by our bodies to create **Vitamin D** which provides **health benefits** that may help ward **off serious illnesses such as** cancer, possibly Covid-19, heart disease — and includes mental benefits such as a boosted mood!

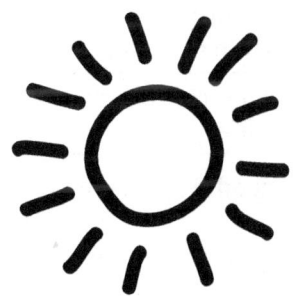

You can become more optimistic, positive and cheerful just by getting a little sun!

Your Emotional Intelligence 10-Minute Test

EQ (emotional quotient) measures emotional intelligence (EI) which is one's ability to be self aware, understand, manage and control their emotions.

Your success in life relies more on EQ than it does IQ (intelligence quotient). The following self-assessment can help you learn your EQ strengths and weaknesses (an unofficial test, but fun to learn!).

> Rank each statement as follows:
> 0 (Never) 1 (Rarely) 2 (Sometimes) 3 (Often) 4 (Always)

Self Awareness	
0 1 2 3 4	My feelings are clear to me at any given moment.
0 1 2 3 4	Emotions play an important part in my life.
0 1 2 3 4	My moods impact the people around me.
0 1 2 3 4	I find it easy to put words to my feelings.
0 1 2 3 4	My moods are easily affected by external events.
0 1 2 3 4	I can easily sense when I'm going to be angry.
0 1 2 3 4	I readily tell others my true feelings.
0 1 2 3 4	I find it easy to describe my feelings.

Self Awareness	
0 1 2 3 4	Even when I'm upset, I'm aware of what's happening to me.
0 1 2 3 4	I am able to stand apart from my thoughts and feelings and examine them.

Self Management	
0 1 2 3 4	I accept responsibility for my reactions.
0 1 2 3 4	I find it easy to make goals and stick with them.
0 1 2 3 4	I am an emotionally balanced person.
0 1 2 3 4	I am a very patient person.
0 1 2 3 4	I can accept critical comments from others without becoming angry.
0 1 2 3 4	I maintain my composure, even during stressful times.
0 1 2 3 4	If an issue does not affect me directly, I don't let it bother me.
0 1 2 3 4	I can restrain myself when I feel anger towards someone.
0 1 2 3 4	I control urges to overindulge in things that could damage my well-being.
0 1 2 3 4	I direct my energy into creative work or hobbies.

Social Awareness	
0 1 2 3 4	I consider the impact of my decisions on other people.
0 1 2 3 4	I can easily tell if people around me are becoming annoyed.

Social Awareness	
0 1 2 3 4	I sense it when a person's mood changes.
0 1 2 3 4	I am able to be supportive when giving bad news to others.
0 1 2 3 4	I am generally able to understand the way other people feel.
0 1 2 3 4	My friends can tell me intimate things about themselves.
0 1 2 3 4	It genuinely bothers me to see other people suffer.
0 1 2 3 4	I usually know when to speak and when to be silent.
0 1 2 3 4	I care what happens to other people.
0 1 2 3 4	I understand when people's plans change.

Social Skills	
0 1 2 3 4	I am able to show affection.
0 1 2 3 4	I am able to manage relationships well.
0 1 2 3 4	I find it easy to share my deep feelings with others.
0 1 2 3 4	I am good at motivating others.
0 1 2 3 4	I am a fairly cheerful person.
0 1 2 3 4	It is easy for me to make friends.
0 1 2 3 4	People tell me I am sociable and fun.
0 1 2 3 4	I like helping people.

Social Skills	
0 1 2 3 4	Others can depend on me.
0 1 2 3 4	I am able to make someone else feel better if they are very upset.

EQ Strengths – Mark your EQ total scores for each category to assess your strengths and areas for improvement.

Category	Score	Total
Self Awareness	0 2 4 6 8 10 12 14 16 18 20 22 24 25 26 28 30 32 34 36 38 40	
Self Management	0 2 4 6 8 10 12 14 16 18 20 22 24 25 26 28 30 32 34 36 38 40	
Social Awareness	0 2 4 6 8 10 12 14 16 18 20 22 24 25 26 28 30 32 34 36 38 40	
Social Skills	0 2 4 6 8 10 12 14 16 18 20 22 24 25 26 28 30 32 34 36 38 40	

Measure your effectiveness in each category using the following key:

0 – 24	Needs attention. Area for Improvement: Multiple Opportunities for Development and Growth
25 – 34	Effective functioning: Consider strengthening
35 – 40	Enhanced skills: EQ is an asset. Use strengths as leverage to develop weaker areas. Be a role model.

Source: Unknown

Get Engaged in the Community – Give back. See how that feels 😊

P.S. It feels great! / P.S.S. Ask your parents, first!

- Donate all the clothes that no longer fit you!
- Consider joining the SDGs Challenge 2021 *SDGsChallenge.org*
- Lend money to an organization like Kiva for businesses in the developing World (Micro loan program) *kiva.org*
- Donate to a local crowd funding project. (There are now over 2,000 sites globally to choose from!)
- Donate to any charity. Here are some global causes:
  - UNICEF **/** *unicef.org*
  - Redcross **/** *redcross.org*
  - Save The Children **/** *savethechildren.org*
  - Green Peace Int. **/***greenpeace.org*
  - Habitat for Humanity **/** *habitat.org*
  - Union of Concerned Scientists **/** *ucsusa.org*
  - One **/** *one.org*
  - Water **/** *water.org*
  - Make a Wish Foundation **/** *wish.org*
- Support global youth teams creating tangible solutions to real world problems! www.SDGsChallenge.org/support-solutions-1

"Know Thyself"

or

"To find yourself, think for yourself."

Socrates

If there was ever a reason to PERK UP!
Consider this:

"A sad soul can kill you quicker, far quicker, than a germ."

John Steinbeck

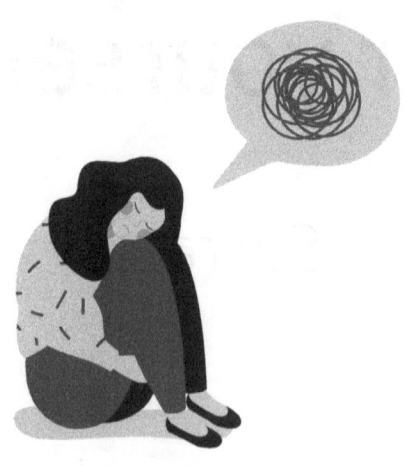

Decided Advantages of Down Time

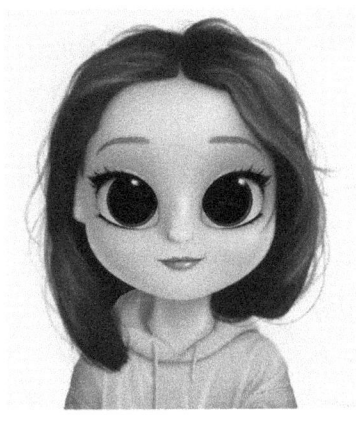

The first days of quarantine were very sad and stressful for me because everything was very new and online school was very difficult . It was strange to talk and interact with a screen and not be with my friends.

When I went out for the first time in quarantine, I was very excited. But when the day finally came it was very good and sad at the same time, because everyone was wearing masks and we couldn't get out of the car. Also, I was very scared because I have heard that a lot of people were dying because of the coronavirus here in Ecuador.

All days I wake up, have school and then I have nothing to do, I only watch TV or look at my phone, but then one day I was thinking and I decided instead of being bored all the time and not doing anything, to take advantage of this situation and do something productive. Since that day I started thinking different and doing lots of different things.

I think it is very important to stay positive in this time that we are in lockdown because we can take advantage of it, we can spend more time with our family and learn more things because we have more time.

Agusta Villalba, 13, Ecuador

Be Creative with Your Money

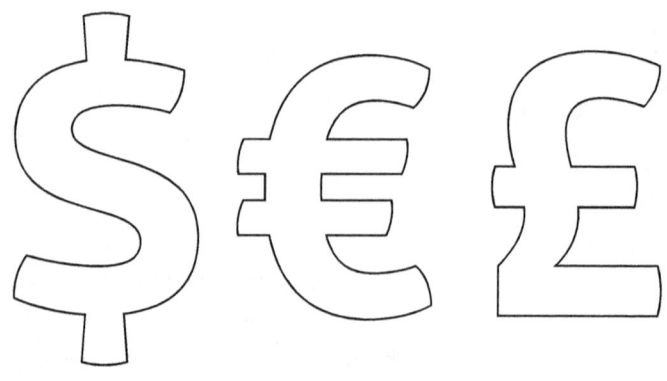

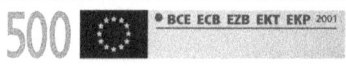

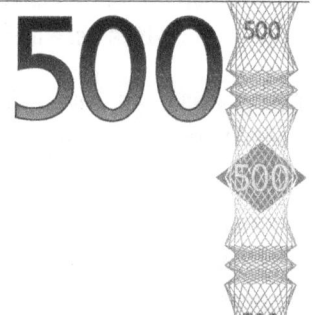

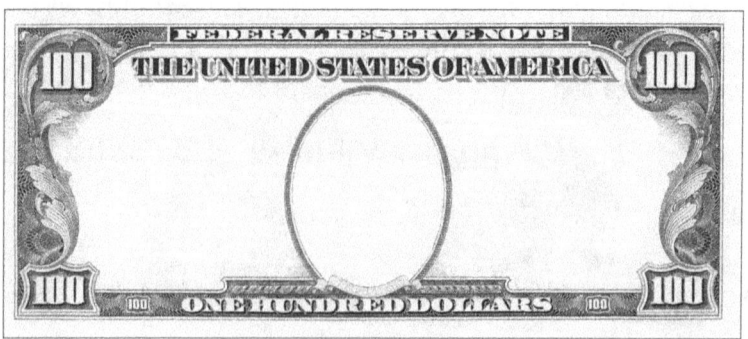

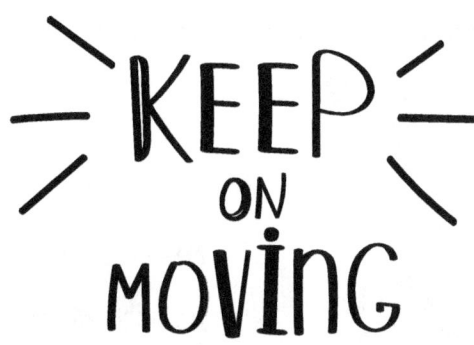

Socially Distanced Activites for Socializing + Mind + Body
BOOST!

(some can be solo)

Chess	Darts
Tennis	Raquet Ball
Volleyball	Pool / Billiards
Yoga	Gym Workout
Kite or Wind surfing	Jet Ski
	Zip line
Crossfit	Snowboarding
Roller Coaster	F1 Go-Carts
Inline Skating / Roller Blading	Board Games
Skateboarding	
Video Games	

The Grace of God

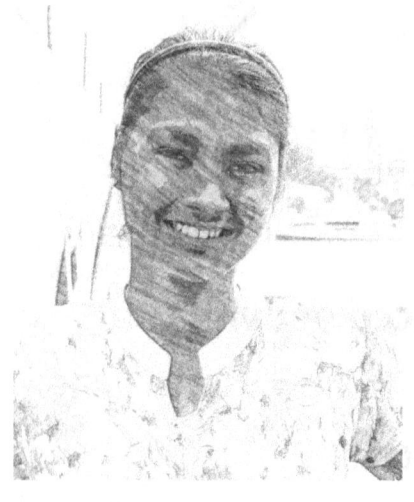

During the lockdown, the movements were restricted.

Initially when we couldn't go to school we felt lonely, however class was connected through virtual mode since starting of the new class we were not able to get the warmth and closeness as in the physical classrooms.

We miss our old friends on a regular basis. I missed direct interaction with my classmates and teachers however, we are at the comfort of our parents and almighty God, what we missed from school was fulfilled by community prayers and phone calls that lifted up our spirit and our life was going in a fruitful manner.

If all these things were locked down, then we would have felt isolation and loneliness but by the grace of God we all were blessed with communication channels and spiritual food for thought and action. Yes, we do have a lot of work pressure, assignments and online submission deadlines.

We were missing the consultative and collaborative efforts on our class work and that burdens and sometimes gives stressful moments.

Gracia Jeniefer, 16, India

Believe in You

P.S.

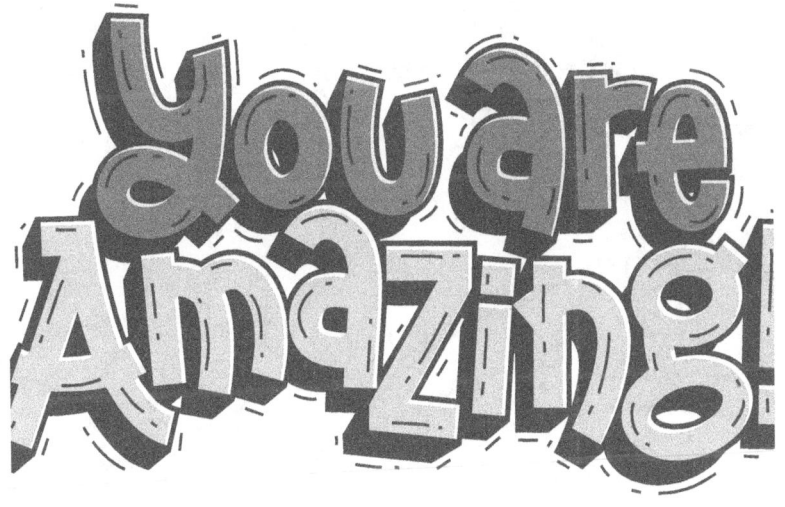

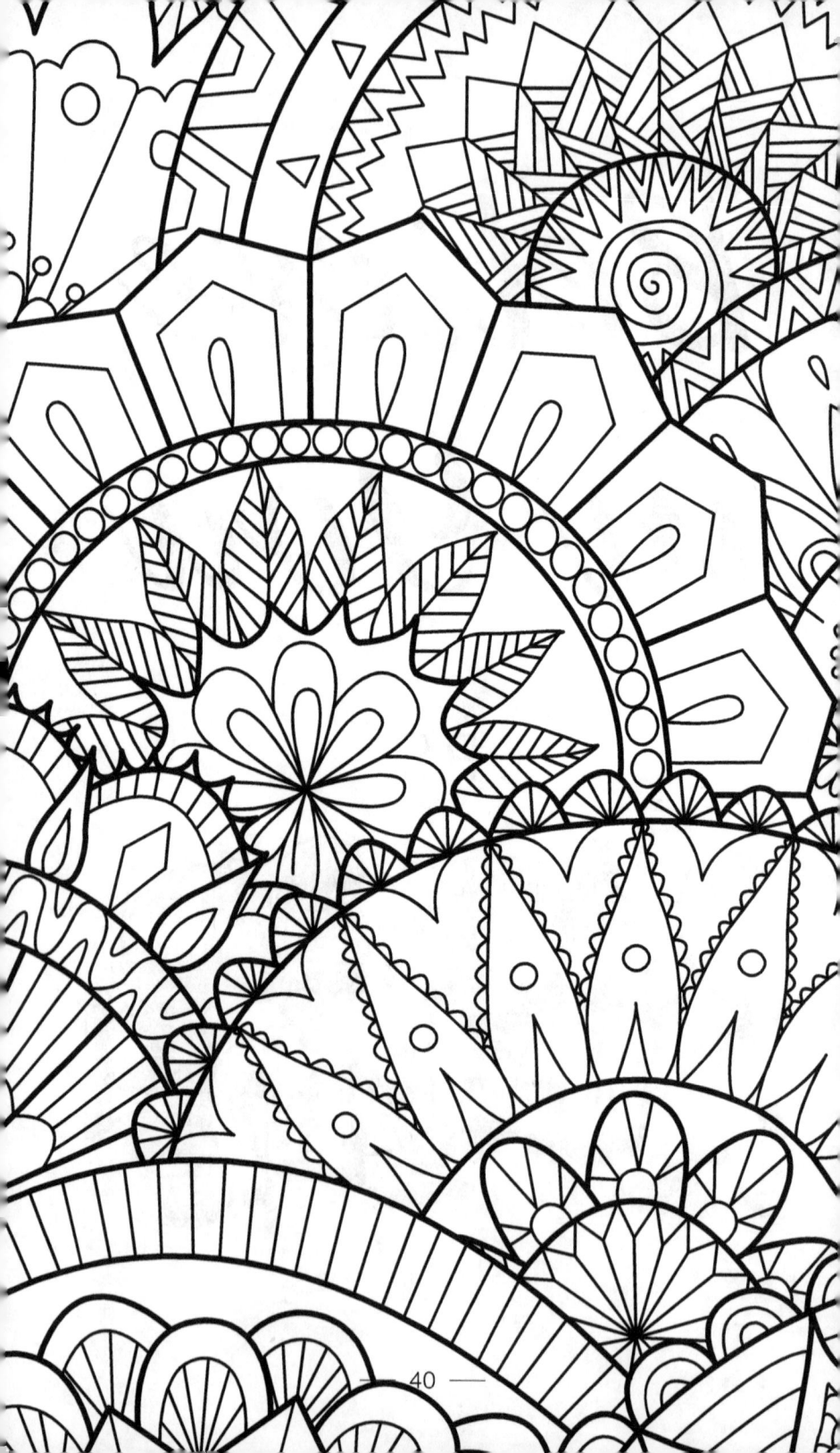

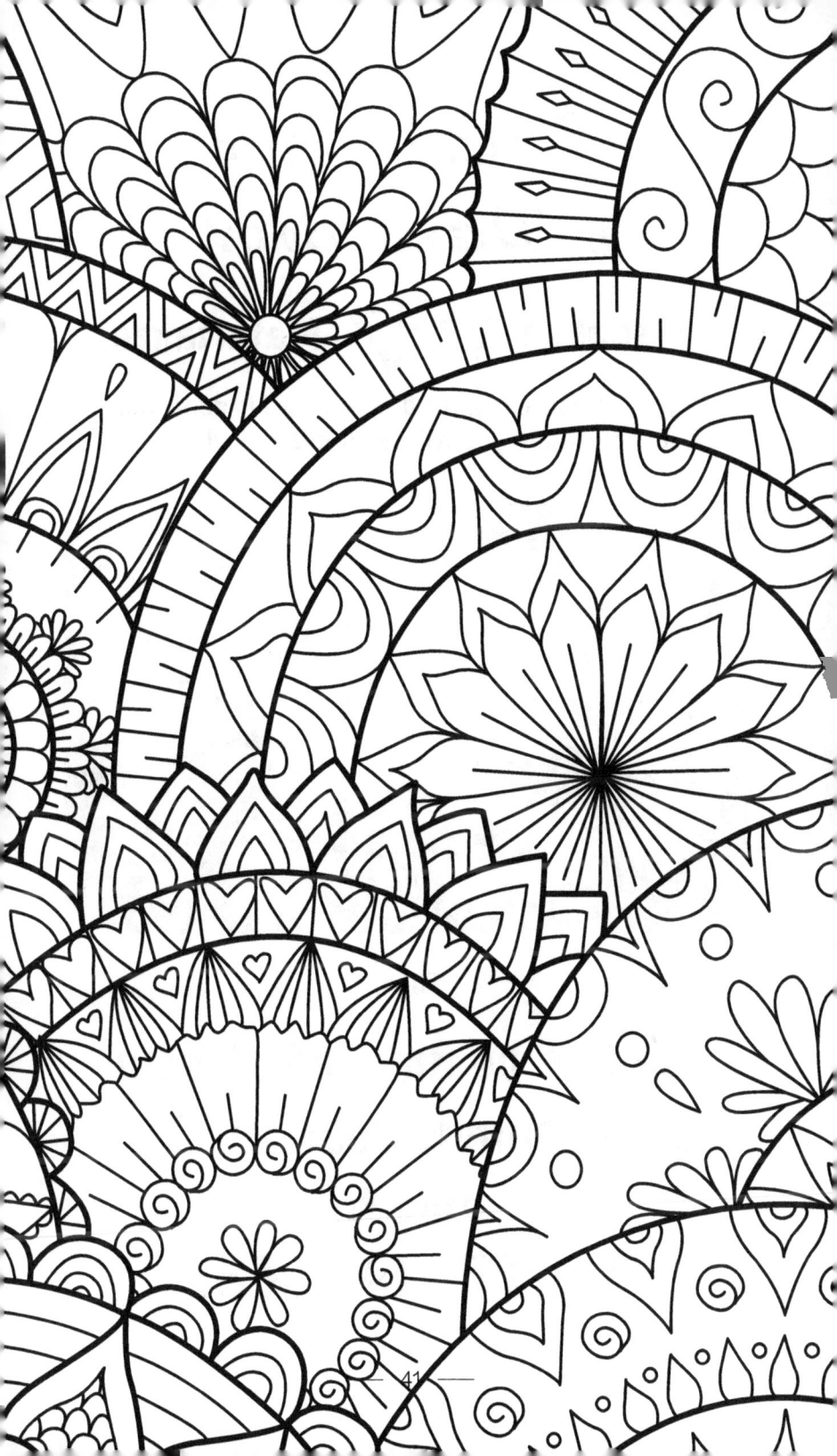

Treasure Map or Dream Board

Visualize ⇒ Materialize!

Once your treasure map or dream board is done, hang or place it somewhere you will see it every day!

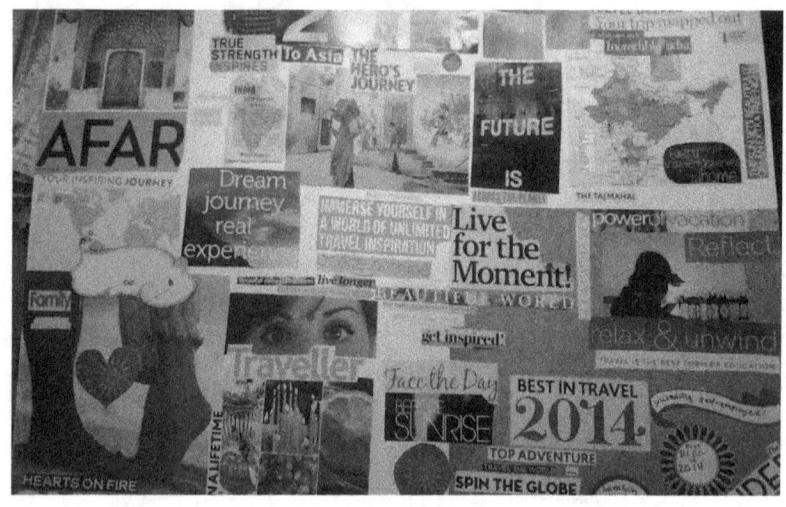

Then,

Wait to be amazed at how many things your mind is able to MATERIALIZE!

Use Treasure Mapping to visualize your dreams and aim to move them toward reality!

WHY? WHAT IS THIS?!

A visual representation of what you aim to attain or achieve in the form of words, images, photos, even things! Helps your brain by providing snapshot of your desires and aspirations! Paste into this book or think BIG and get some poster board! You can experiment in this book in the meantime.

WHAT DO YOU NEED?

- Magazines or newspapers you don't mind destroying
- Scissors
- Glue stick (ideal as it's less messy and you can move things around before fully dries!)

HOW TO DO IT?

1. Consider your theme or just start flipping through pages to hunt for words, concepts, things that resonate for you, ideas that you find alluring for your life or that reinforce your current, near, or long term plans and dreams.
2. Start clipping things out!
3. Paste into the next few pages (or that poster board!) and arrange as you like.

Treasure Map or Dream Board

Paste
images of
dreams
here!

Treasure Map it!
My Career & Future Work plans

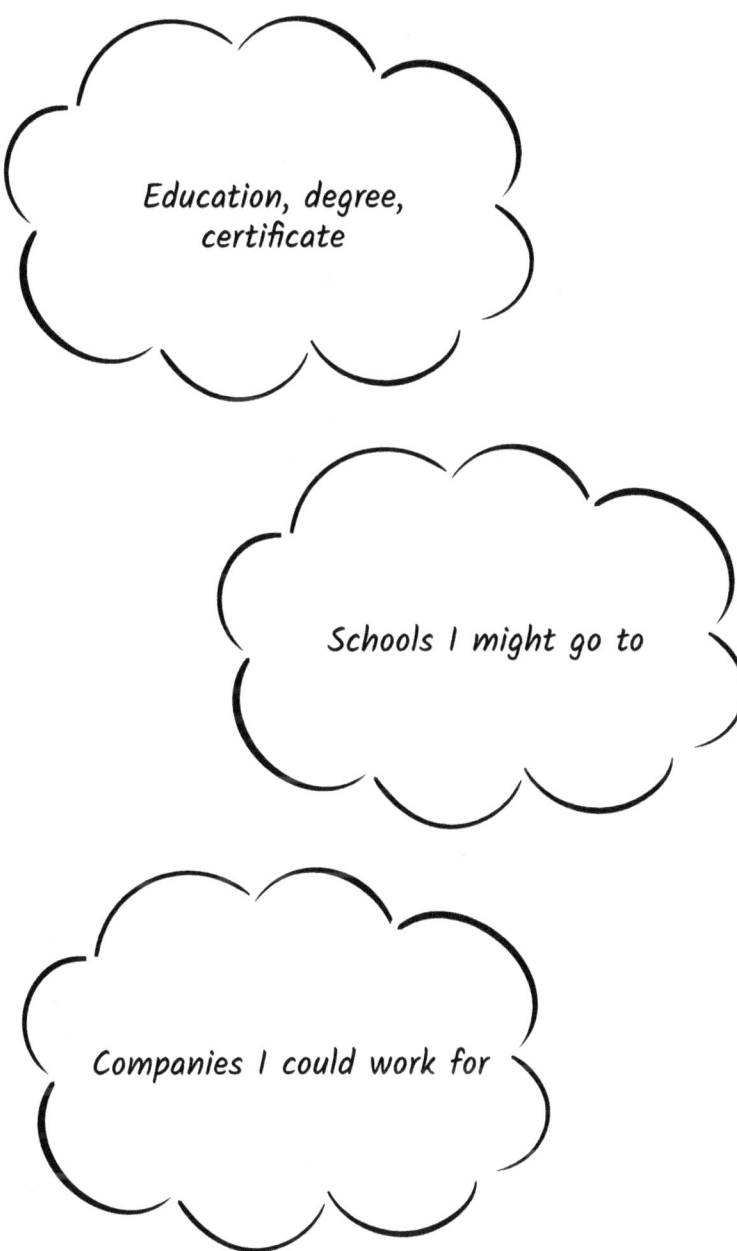

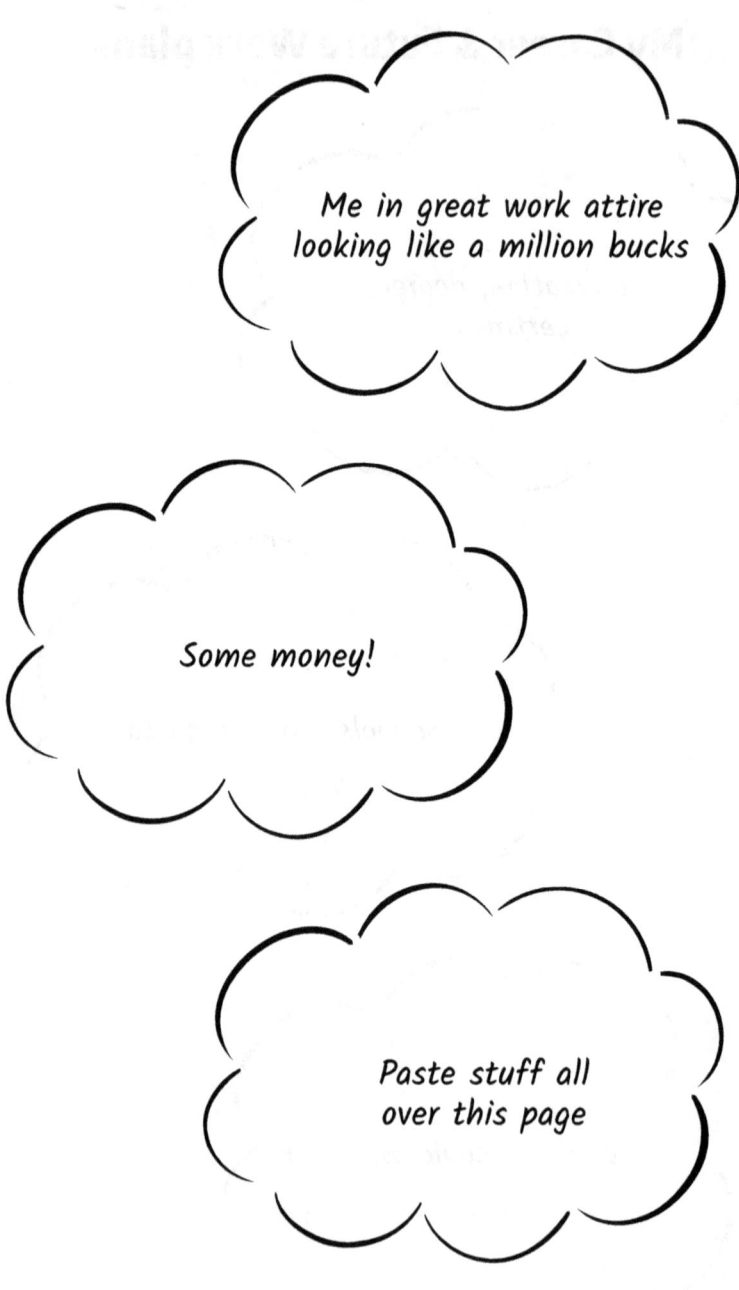

More TOLERANCE, please!
Not everyone has to agree with or think like you, for you to be okay.

Keep an open mind.

"Variety is the spice of life"

You are entitled to your own thoughts and opinions and SO ARE OTHERS!

BE KIND.

To find harmony, keep judgements to a minimum.

Proven Mood Boosters

- Volunteer at a local charity - if you can safely.

- Spend down-time making a collage of favorite photos (physical, paper based photos, remember those?!). Display so you see happy memories every day.

- Create a "Treasure Map". Cut out words, pictures, and other items from magazines or newspapers that project a future you. Your mind will help you work toward becoming or attaining it –and you won't even 'know' it!

- Think about all you're grateful for and make a cheat sheet you can keep handy.

- Write a letter to your future self about how you're feeling right now. Hide in a place where you'll find it one day to further reflect.

- Meditate or practice Yoga, Tai-chi or even Feng shui!...

- Re-arrange, paint or (re)decorate your bedroom.

- Take a hot bubble bath!

- Go for a long, leisurely walk or hike.

- Swim!

Life Flows On

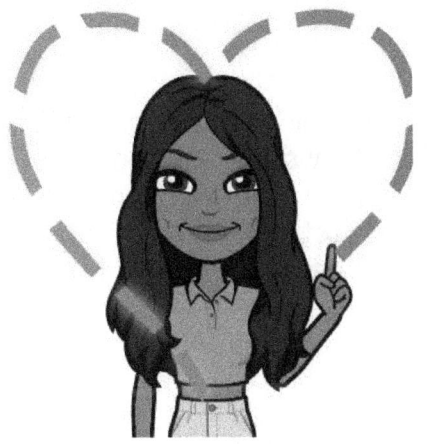

This whole entire experience has been quite an interesting time for me.

I believe I definitely got lucky with having more privileges then some, being able to remain in isolation, doing my own thing, not needing to support any family members or being in a toxic household like others. But even with my luck, these past few months have been an on-going roller-coaster of emotions.

I have noticed a big divide between people during this time, where many thrive and others dive into a dark hole. Where we all feel unmotivated, lost, confused, scared, or even all around miserable.

Then there are others who got to share their creativity during this time, start businesses, branch out into new hobbies, etc. I believe I am in a weird area of both. Every single day I have felt constantly unmotivated and burnt out, and numb to the sadness of having to go through another day wondering when we will be able to go back to "normal" (which is most likely not in a long while, especially in the USA).

While having to still deal with the switch to virtual learning with our very awkward meeting calls and having our older teachers yelling at us for feeling uncomfortable for going on mute or not showing our face, we had to watch our national cases of corona continue to rise and see people protesting to coronavirus.

The first few months resulted in a lot of stress, worry, and disappointment. My mother is a teacher so I had to go help her immediately clean out her whole entire classroom within only a few days.

My parents and I spent weeks planning a home graduation for my sister and cousin since they sadly could not have a proper one. I occasionally did have to go to school and work for my student council in order to set up senior activities and a graduation drive-by, and even while that was one of the more fun events that occurred during this virus, I was so scared to even be within a few feet of my closest friends that I had to work alongside with.

With all of these activities I still had to study for classes, got into debates about the current Black Lives Matter movement, have my boyfriend of nearly a year break up with me, and just feel like I all around had no purpose. When everything bad basically hit me in mid-July, I was mentally exhausted and felt stuck. I decided that I needed to change that.

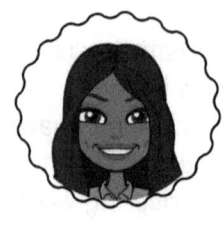

I went on a rampage of changing my living space and myself. Meaning I painted my room, rearranged it, cut my hair, started learning new hairstyles, workout, etc. I did things that would keep me both busy but also help me mentally (the new arrangements of my room cleared my head and made everything feel seem more organized).

I decided to reach out to my friends and practice talking to them more, communicating with others during this time so both of us would feel like they weren't alone through all of this.

I started learning how to drive! I used to be terrified of that but I decided to face my fear and now I love being able to drive

aimlessly in my car and go new places without worrying about getting in contact with others. I believe trying all these new things or hobbies and reaching out to those I usually wouldn't have, has definitely helped me out during this time.

I also have been working closely in my Teens Dream Mental Health Hub, a collaborative of teens working to build projects surrounding mental health awareness, and it has helped me a lot to have open conversations about mental health during meetings and within projects or webinars.

Overall, I've been trying to take everything day by day - even though it seems everyday is blending together. I try to find something new to look forward to every new day and just remind myself that soon, we will get out of this. I'm not sure how long that will be, but I have hope that we will.

Ryann Chalmers, USA

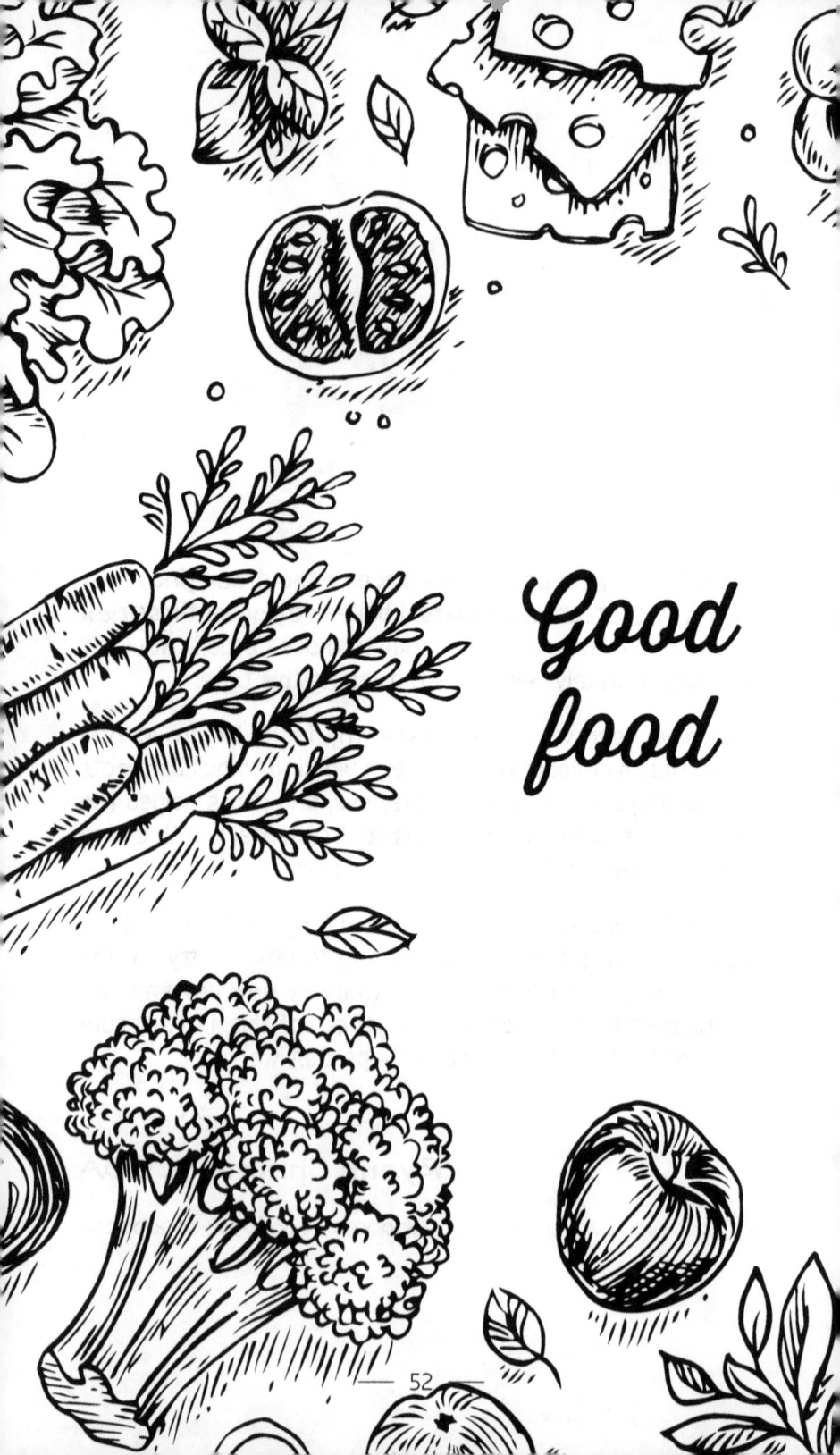

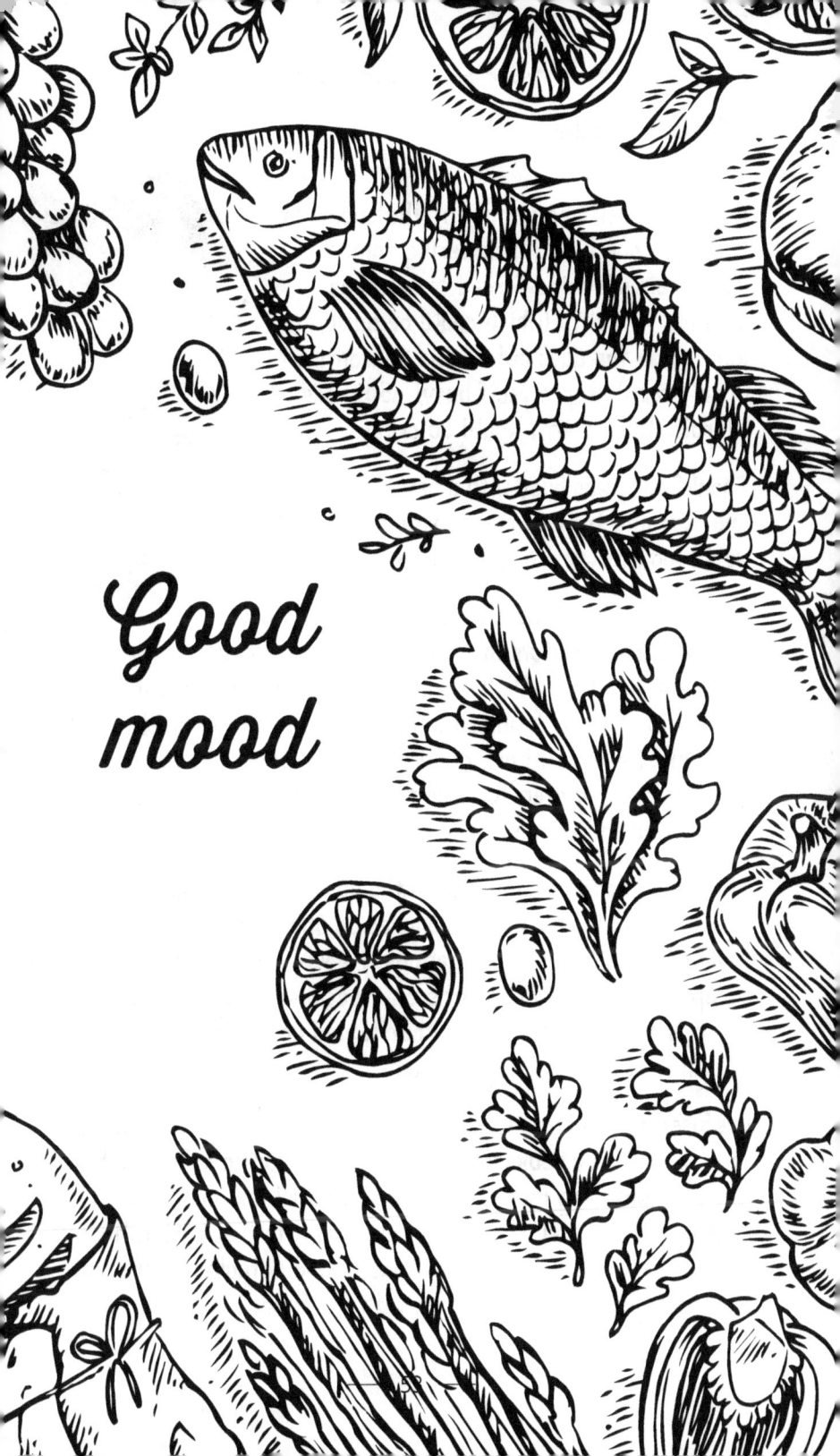

Close Calls

As a teenager who is only at that point in life when she keeps discovering things about herself, being forced to be alone with my thoughts (which could be easily ignored on the days before the quarantine when I could keep myself busy) now made me literally think that I would go crazy.

Thankfully, I was busy with a new theatre project and learning Italian, the only two things that I would look forward to for the days to come.

Other than that, I would sometimes spend hours on Instagram, watching videos or memes, which made me hate myself. Instagram makes me become an addict, to the point when I can't physically stop myself from scrolling. However, at one point during the quarantine I was able to make the big step towards the healing of my addiction and uninstalled Instagram.

Still, what I recall the most from the quarantine time is the hours I would spend in bed, with earphones on and watching the ceiling, trying to understand my feelings. I would not talk to anybody except my family (and that's only because I was forced to). I would just ignore the friends that texted or called me because I wouldn't feel like talking to them.

I refused to read anything, which is strange enough as I usually read some of the books in one sitting, even during school nights. Not even watching movies or series tempted me anymore. I was really down and I felt like I didn't even want to feel better. It was very hard to drop that phase I was in and actually start doing more things and regain contact with my friends.

At that point, I entered a state in which the only thing that kept me sane was making plans for after the quarantine.

I talked with all my close or not that close friends and arranged meetings with them. I talked a lot through texts and calls with a classmate of mine, who is now one of my best friends. We shared the things we went through during quarantine and a lot more, which brought us closer.

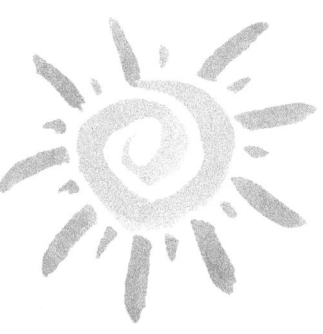

When I think about it now, I consider myself lucky that I had someone listening to me rant during quarantine. He helped me regain my mental stability and I like to think that I helped him too.

That's why my advice would be: ask for help. Don't go through anything alone, because it's so much harder to keep being balanced. And always keep your friends close.

Sofia Bacanu, 17, Romania

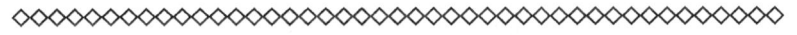

What do you think of this?!

"No human thing is of serious importance."
Plato

Reminds us of

"This too shall pass"

which really only means...

"It is the mark of an educated mind to be able to entertain a thought without accepting it."

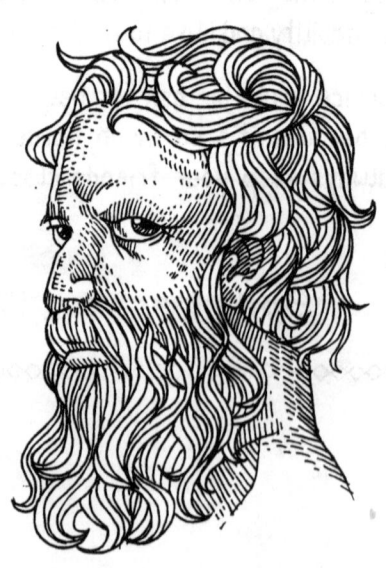

Time Out!

What size shoe do you wear?
_____

How many pandemics have you lived through?
_____

REMEMBER How old you were when you lost your first tooth?

What nickname do you call your mother?

How often do you CALL your mother?

What day is it today?
_____
What time did you wake up? _____
How much do you weigh? Bit personal? Okay, forget it.

What color is your car?
_____
No car? How do you get to work?
_____
No work? What's your hobby?
_____

Ask a question here that you've always wondered about
_____
_____

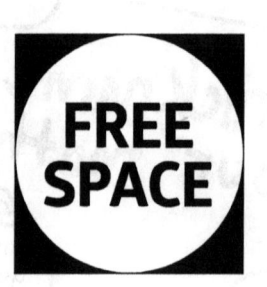

Put your pet's paw print here

Making the Most of a Holding Pattern

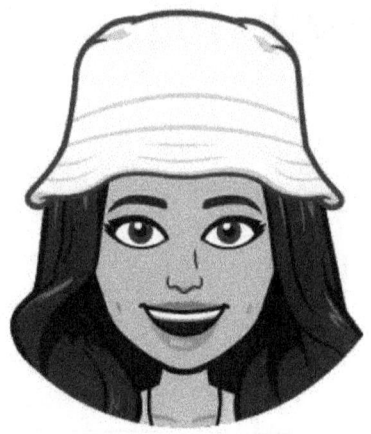

I stopped counting what day of lockdown it is, and stopped counting the number of weeks in week 7. Then, almost two months of lockdown. Level 4. Meaning we couldn't even exit the house, and if we did so, a penalty fee awaited us.

I am currently living in New Zealand with my best friend. Her family was kind enough to take me home with them, since my family lives all the way in Austria, Europe. Well, to be exact, my dad and my brother do, my mom works in New York and my oldest brother goes to university in Singapore.

I met my friend in boarding school and her family treats me like one of their own and has made me feel welcome like no other.

Many months previously, me and my friend had booked a flight to New York from New Zealand. New York is her dream destination and since my mom worked over there, I invited here to come with me — a long awaited trip to see my family to have the time of my life in the city that never sleeps with my friend!

By mid-February, cases were being reported in Thailand, the US, Australia, Japan and Italy, and the NZ government gradually increased border restrictions, banning flights and banning internationals, such as me, to pass through New Zealand's borders.

What freaks me out, is not knowing when I will see my family next. Even though I have a lovely family by my side, I miss my own. I've endured by spending most of my time with a phone pressed to my ear, alternating between uncontrolled tears and coherent, rational discussion.

Still, I couldn't be grateful enough!

Vivien Dimitrov, 15, New Zealand

◇◇

THROW A ZOOM Dance Party

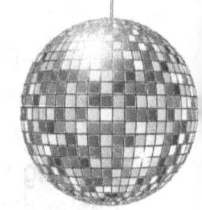

1. Make an invitee list of your fun friends

2. Be creative and make a theme
   (Music genre or costumes?! Or?!)

3. Ask each friend to send you 1, 2, 3 of their favorite tunes

4. Que up all the music
   (Use or make some new D.J. skills)

5. Send over the video meeting link (i.e. zoom, etc) (you may need to subscribe zoom if more than 40min!)

6. Get out some pent-up energy, get some exercise!

ENJOY!

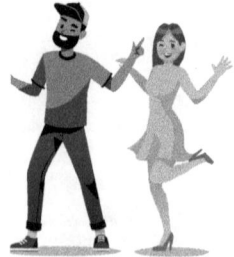
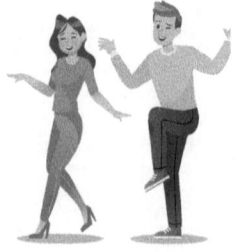

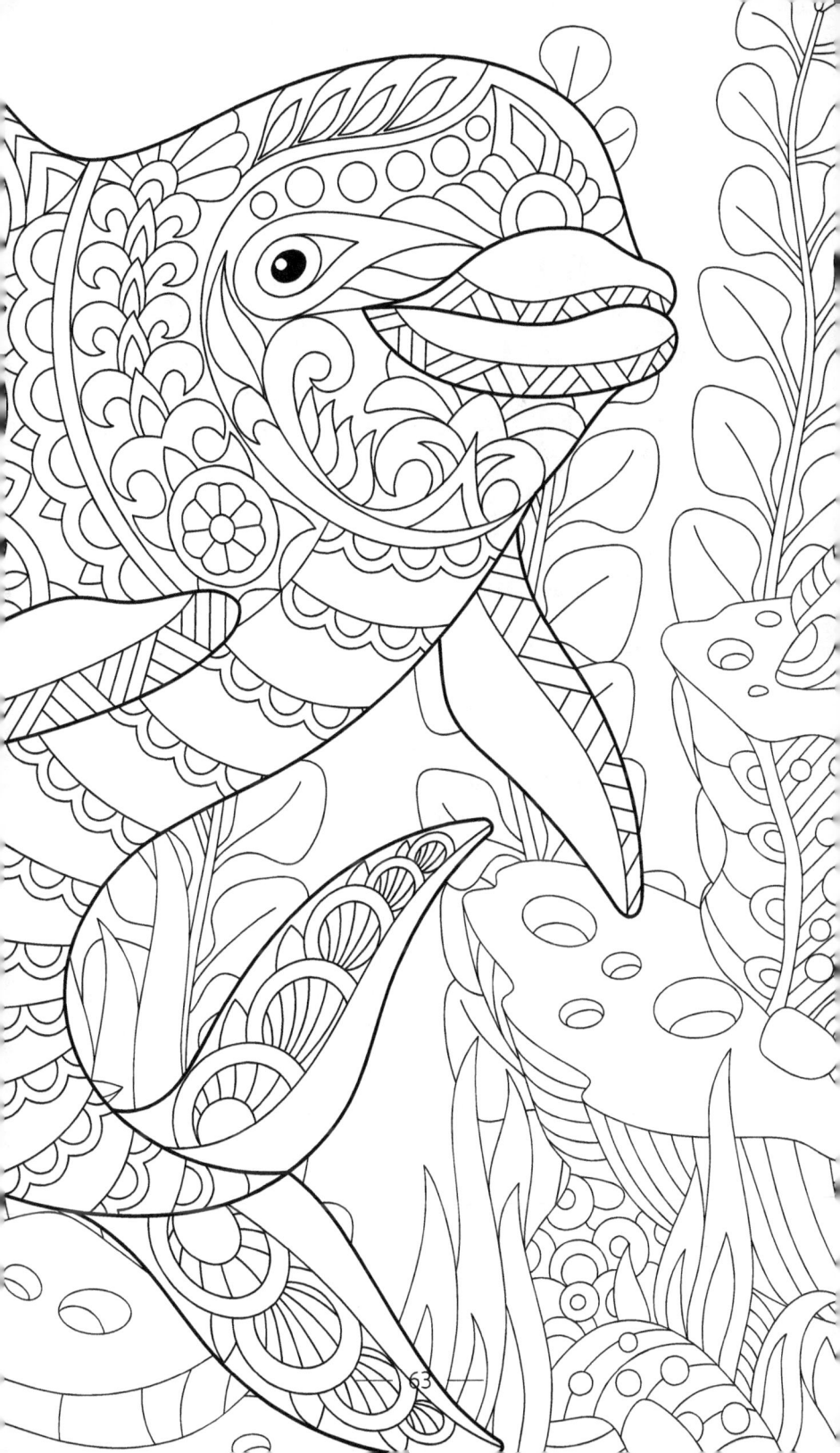

Life Changes

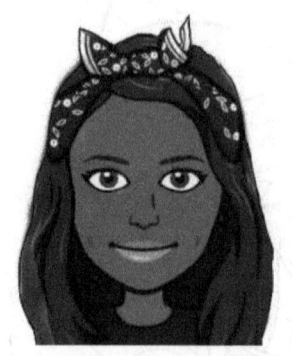

Fitia Robson, 14, Madagascar

Every morning, me and my brother had to wake up at 7:00 am to prepare for school. Starting by getting dressed and eating breakfast. After our morning routine was done, we could now leave the house and wait for our buses.

We arrived at school at 7:40 am and gathered with our friends waiting for the bell to ring. All the students had to follow the school's rules, changing class every 45 min minutes until 3:00 PM. During those 8 hours we could see our teachers and have all kinds of social interactions.

Nowadays, we are stuck at home waking up at whatever time we want and sleeping at whatever time we want since there is no school. When we go out, we are forced to wear a mask. That includes going to the mall, walking in the street and going to the grocery store: basically any public area.

We weren't ready to not go to school for 4 months and school was a big change having to learn through a computer and talk to our teachers through zoom conferences and emails. We also couldn't see our friends and family which means not a lot of social interactions and not a lot of fun.

Online school wasn't harder than normal school, we just had to be more independent and organized, making time for each assignment and tests even though there was a lot.

Quarantine took a lot from everyday life but also created new types of activities to get out of the boredom of being stuck at home.

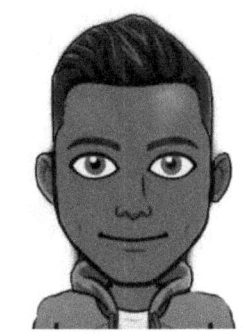

Aro Robson, 15, Madagascar

But we could spend more time with our family than before.

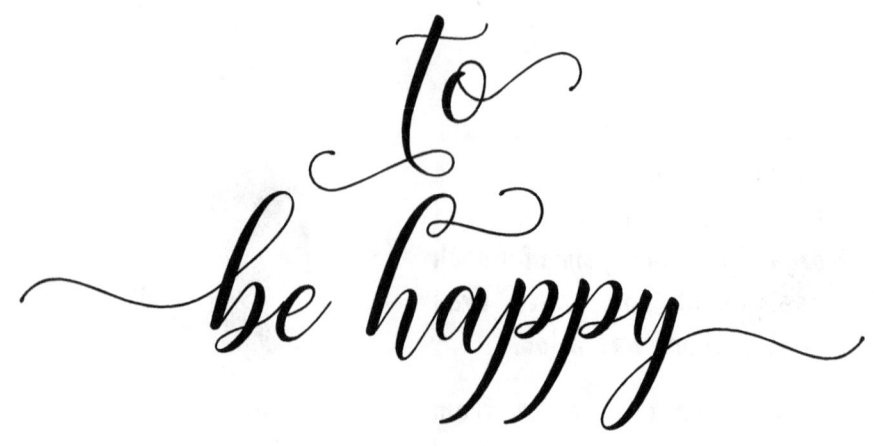

it's not a secret

Keep happy thoughts in mind!

They say:
"Count your blessings'
"Be grateful"
"It's fortunate that..."
"You're so lucky"

Take those things to heart

INTERRUPTING THIS BOOK FOR A SPECIAL (MAYBE CONTROVERSIAL) ANNOUNCEMENT:

ACTIVISM can be a slippery slope from mild **PROTESTING** to more extreme **MARTYRDOM**

ARGUING, FIGHTING, FRUSTRATION. BE CAREFUL

DON'T LET YOUR CAUSES LEAD TO AN UNHAPPY LIFE
THINK ABOUT WHAT YOU REALLY AIM TO ACCOMPLISH

PERHAPS CONSIDER PURPOSEFUL BUT LESS INTENSE:

SOCIAL ENTERPRISE/ ENTREPRENEUR
CHAMPION
ADVOCATE
SOCIAL IMPACT
CHANGEMAKER
CHEERLEADER

Finding the New Comfort Zone

My life has always been a fairly busy one, but with this time to slow down a bit, I have been able to relearn lessons I was taught but did not fully internalize, to pay more attention and devote more time to myself, and do a bit of mental spring cleaning! Having been stuck at home for over half a year I gained a lot! I surprisingly made quite a few positive strides in the right direction with regards to personal growth.

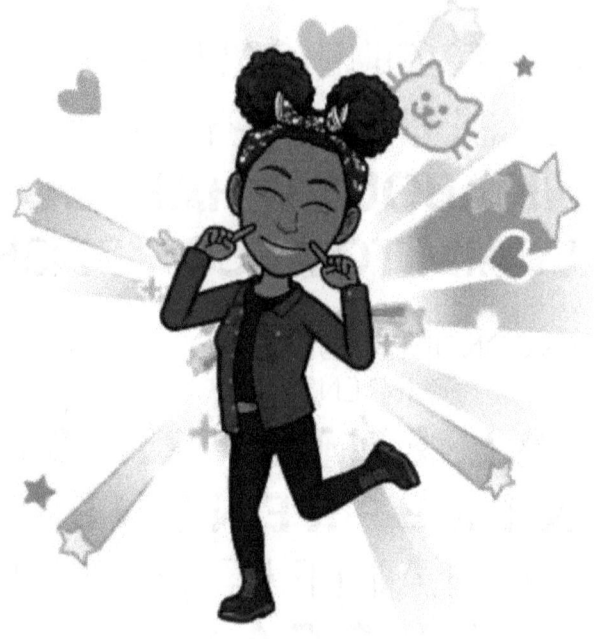

The beginning did not seem oh so promising to say the least. Towards the end of my last year of high school and near the date of my IGCSE finals, there had to be an emergency closure of school on account of the increasing corona cases worldwide. Even though Lesotho did not have a single confirmed case at that time, everything was shut down and scheduled to continue virtually.

Less than two weeks after that, my finals got cancelled! The CIE decided that it was not safe for the students and invigilators alike to stuff themselves in a room for however long for these examinations. Unlike a good number of my peers.

I was devastated! I viewed my IGCSE finals as a chance for me to prove to not only my teachers and my parents, but to myself, just how hard I had been working in preparation for these exams.

The idea of having grades calculated, forecasted and predicted instead of actually writing the papers made me feel as though I was being handed my completion certificate without actually putting in the work.

The first month or two I sat at home contemplating the emptiness of my days. Lamenting the monotony of waking up everyday just to sit around and go back to sleep - the next night having accomplished nothing.

With no consistent routine and nothing to look forward to the next day, sleep became a torturous task. And not too long after that, even getting out of bed in the morning became difficult. I mean what for!? Why wake up if everyday is the exact same meaningless, repetitive nonsense?

I became desperate to the leave the enclosing walls of my bedroom and go out to breathe the air that everyone else was breathing, despite the idea of the coronavirus lingering in the air. It was not even the fact that I missed anyone in particular, but being this normally vibrant, loud and talkative youngling who had not been able to be that ball of energy with friends, I turned to my family. They did not seem interested so one-sided conversation followed another and eventually being around family became very difficult and made me quite anxious. I needed to get out!

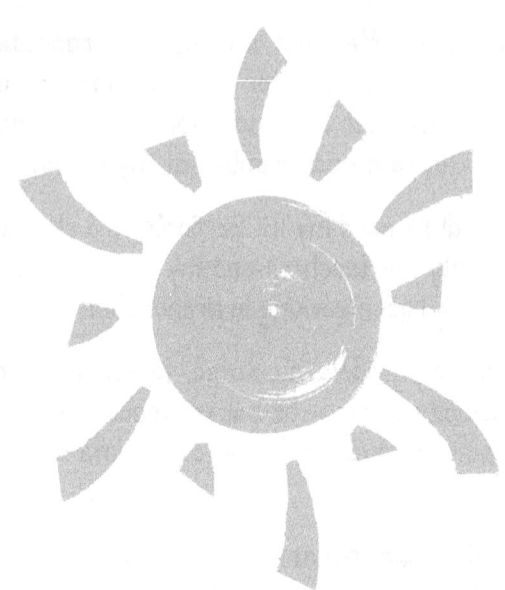

And eventually I did. After many long weeks I was able to somehow convince my mother to allow me to tag along to go do the groceries and boy did I feel great after!

A few more visits to the outside world were exactly what the doctor ordered. I was feeling lighter and happier in no time. Knowing that everything was fairly normal outside of my home I was more at ease and able to spend time on getting myself back to normal.

I invested my time in things I thought could preoccupy my mind, and also rid myself of relationships no longer beneficial. During quarantine I learned and become more comfortable with myself, my future and the world I am currently living in, more than I think I may have been able to learn outside of quarantine.

I adopted new life skills and was able to bring myself closer to the image of what I want to be in life with regards to my faith, physically, emotionally, mentally and academically. I got the chance to figure out what I like, what I do not like and what I plan to do about all of it. I developed philosophies to live by and healthy practices to exercise.

I acquired patience, acceptance, appreciation, overall happiness and serenity because of the uncomfortable and stressful position I have been put in and I think I am better for it!

I used to see it all over social media but was never able to relate its truth to my own life. Having been given the opportunity to watch the people around me flourishing; from starting YouTube channels, to investing in their futures, and developing pages and websites to exhibit the things that they are passionate about, I can now agree in the belief that the lockdown has been a blessing in disguise.

It has allowed everyone a little time to themselves – to reevaluate, to rethink and possibly reconnect with others near, and far.

Even though I have already grown drastically, I am still growing and am tremendously excited for the journey ahead!

Neo Mokhakala, 17, Lesotho

Change Your Thoughts & You Change Your World

Design your unique mask

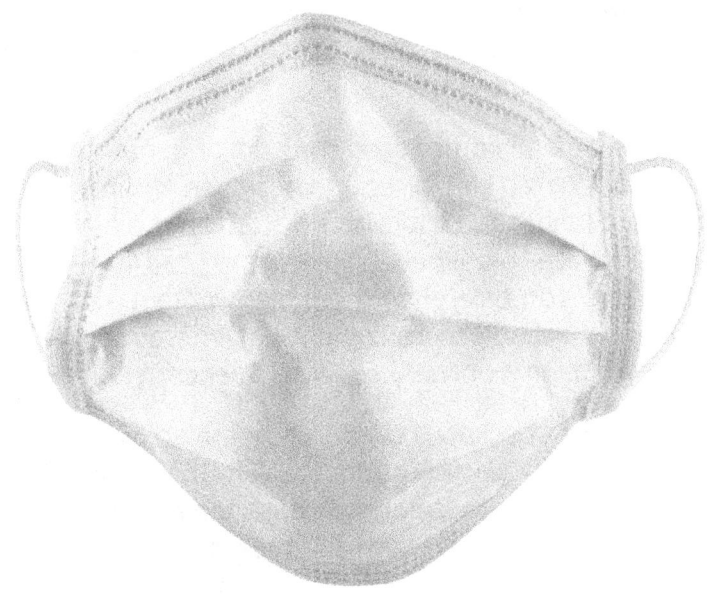

Leap of Faith

I thought that 2020 would be a great year (a wonderful leap year) that would bring me joy and happiness. However, I could never imagine the wild turn it would take. It shocked me to see the entire world go into lockdown. For the first time in my life, everything was shut, there were no malls, no restaurants, no parks, nothing open at all.

Everyone was at home, scared of getting infected by the virus. I just hated the experience of spending my daily life surrounded by four walls with no friends at all. My school shifted its base to online lectures where I had to sit in front of a laptop for three hours per day without my friends. Normally in school, there is plenty of interaction but now since everything is online there is zero per cent of it available.

During breaks at school, I used to play and enjoy myself with my friends but now I only get to speak to them through voice and video calls, which is boring. I miss the fun we had in our good old days, everyone used to crack jokes and share their meals during the break. COVID-19 has brought a lot of ups and downs in my life. It has separated me from my friends but at the same allowed me to reflect on my actions. It has taught me to be self-reliant.

I can proudly say that I know how to cook and feed myself. I know how to solve various Rubix cubes that once seemed difficult. This all has been a substitute for my squad, my friends, whom I will never forget.

Dhruv D'Souza, 13, India

Don't forget to Be awesome

Cultivate Positive Emotions
(negative ones are humbug)

- Get outside! Fresh air does wonder for the mind + spirit.
- Choose a relatively quiet location and look up at the sky. Ponder its expansiveness.
- Consider all that's good in your life.
- Make yourself a picnic lunch and go to your favorite spot with a friend, social distance, of course...

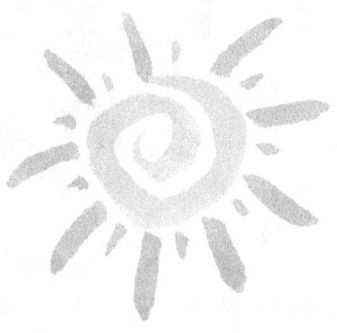

- Buy a green plant - if you can commit to watering it regularly (dead plants don't cultivate positive emotions).
- Buy some flowers. Take a big whiff, take in their beauty.
- Better yet, pick some flowers (just not from your neighbors yard).

- Push any negative emotions OUT of your mind as soon as they enter and REPLACE with uplifting thoughts.
- Write down and rehearse positive messages (affirmations). Recite to yourself daily. Believe in yourself.
- Look in the mirror and smile big as you say "I'm awesome!"
- Trust yourself. Embrace optimism.
- Create a garden and watch it come to life and grow. (Again, the watering thing).
- Go for a mask-less walk in nature, alone and enjoy the peace, serenity and again, FRESH AIR! Deep breaths! No Phone.

Coping with Covid

Get Moving

Consistent motion is the surest way to keep your bodily functions working properly and body weight in check. Aerobic exercises such as walking, running, stepping, bicycling, swimming and even cleaning! dancing and gardening each stimulates your heart muscles, amp up your metabolism and promotes the flow of oxygen through increased blood circulation - all great for a healthy heart. Physical exercise works wonders for your mental state and studies have shown it also improves brain function, reduces stress, anxiety and improves the mood.

Express Yourself & Take Action

If your circumstances are getting you down or if you are feeling tired or simply find you need to make a change, positive forward action will move you along toward more productive and positive headspace and diminsh any noise inside you mind. Anxiety is a vicious circle of thoughts that circulate within your mind. Express yourself better, let the thoughts flow and translate them into action.

Return to Nature

Add herbs to your daily routine and diet. Herbs are all natural and help heal while also connect you to the Earth. There are many herbs that can be used to relieve health issues - for instance for tension try lavender oil, for depression try St. John's Wort and for peace of mind and relaxation try a hot cup of chamomile or green tea.

Create

Consider a creative activity that will keep you engaged and by default this will alleviate unwanted thoughts from entering your mind. Consider the things that you enjoy or find a new hobby. The idea is to leave no time in your life to ruminate on bad vibes.

Meditate

Meditation is an age old practice - literally an art that promotes greater health and wellbeing and consists of clearing your mind and finding inner quiet and peace. It is useful as it keeps the forces in your life and body in balance and helps build a sense of wellbeing by providing synchronization. By meditating you may likely find you have greater control.

Inspirational advice credited to Muhammad Anas Virk, Young Business Entrepreneur and Blogger, Pakistan

Keep Calm and Carry On

Due to the COVID-19 pandemic, a lot has changed for me. Throughout the school year and summertime, I was going to participate in multiple events outside of Taiwan, however, they were all canceled due to travel restrictions.

I felt that all my hard work and effort to prepare for these events were for nothing and I am not really sure when everything will go back to normal. Also, due to the conflict between Taiwan and China, I feel many uncertainties about my future.

All these factors have brought stress upon me, which made me lose hope. Despite everything that is happening around me, I have tried to remain calm and appreciate everything that I still have. I talk to my friends and family about what I stress about which allows me to feel a sense of serenity.

Some other ways I relieve my stress include playing my viola, drawing, playing golf, and other activities that help me relax. With all the uncertainties surrounding us, I think that sometimes it is really important to take a step back, relax, and take it day by day.

Katie Chu, 15, Taiwan

Take 5 minutes
uninterrupted not distracted
just focused and present

Breath in Inhale

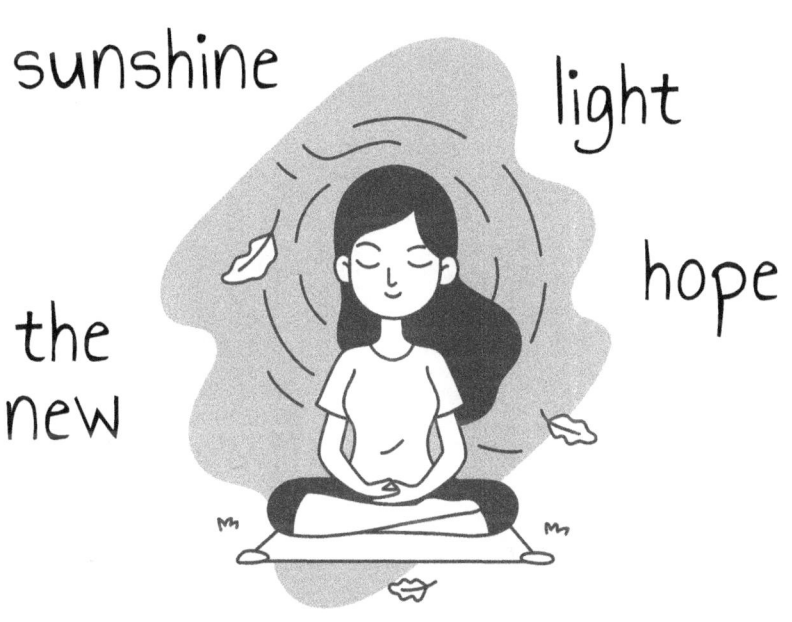

sunshine

light

the new

hope

happiness

Exhale!

Repeat after me, out loud:

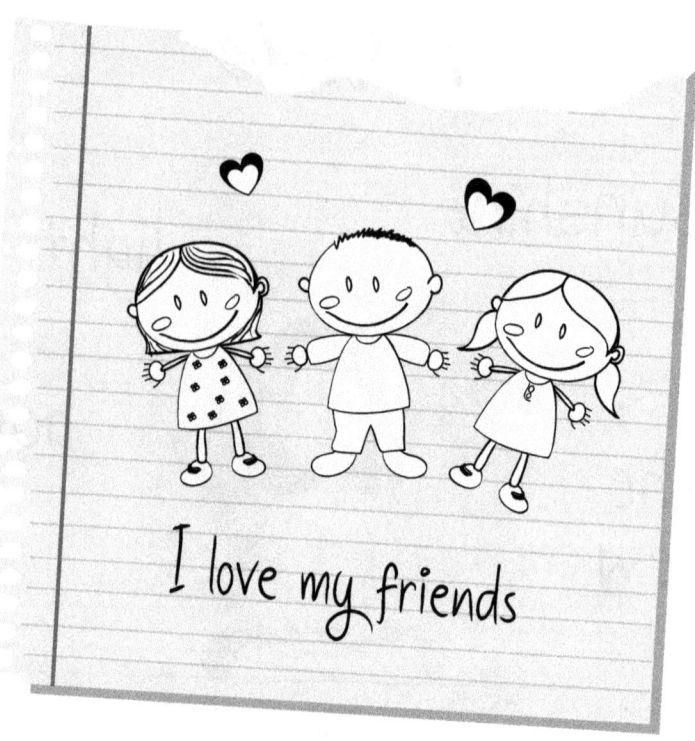

Even though you may not be able to hang-out call one if you're in need of a pick-me-up. Social relationships do wonders for warding off depression. And, this pandemic is a total downer. Friend up.

Who are you?
I am....

(draw some diagrams and pics)

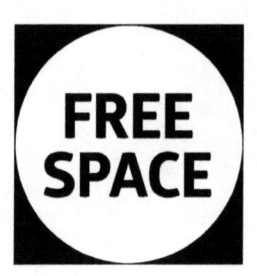

Dip your knuckles in something

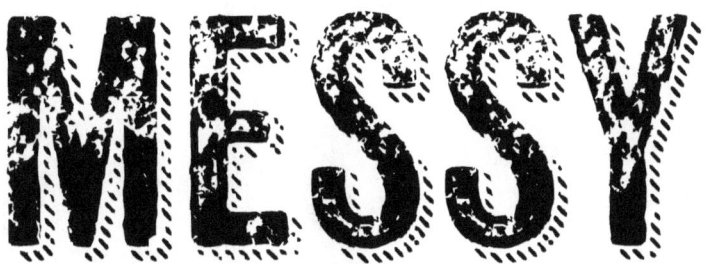

make an imprint here

Time for a break & some Music therapy!

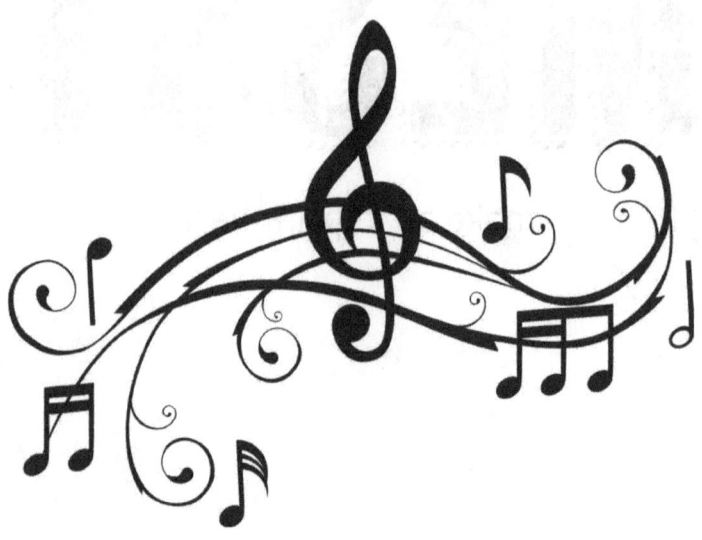

1. find a place with total privacy

2. find a favorite tune

3. sing out loud as if you are on stage

Singing out loud is a great way to alleviate stress and feel happy at the same time.

Fitness or weight loss your thing?

Here are some great apps to try that help you track:

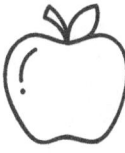 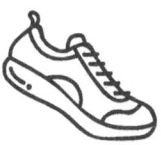 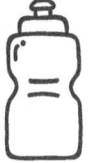

Calories / Food Intake   Steps / exercise daily   Water intake

 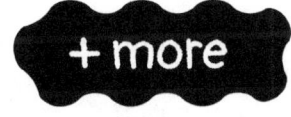

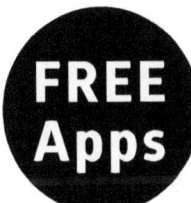

Over 200 to choose from!

- MoniterYourWeight
- Lose It - Fit Now
- Approvo
- NOOM
- Weight Calendar
- MyFitnessPal
- Strava

FREE Apps

Emotional Victory

April 2020
Dear future grandchildren,

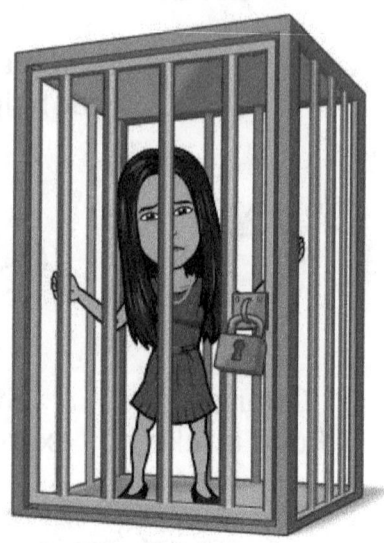

It has been a month since I stepped out of my house. I thought that this situation would just be a joke, something that would dwindle away with time before I would have to go back to junior college to take my final exams. (Although, I was happy that my exams were postponed.)

My day used to be packed with college, activities, classes, studies and play. I took those wonderful days for granted. I took my normal life for granted. I am now very bored.

I feel like a caged bird, trapped and cornered. This is not a pleasant feeling! It is making me overthink. When will I be able to go out again?

With love,
An overthinking Nikki.

May 2020
Dear future curious grandchildren,

Two months have gone by. The COVID cases in Mumbai are increasing rapidly, and Dad (your great-grandfather) is very strict, forbidding me to step out of our two bedroom flat. This is so irritating. Tempers are flaring, and everyone at home seems to be sitting on a ticking bomb of anger and frustration.

With love,
A frustrated Nikki.

June 2020
Dear future super curious grandchildren,

I am sure you assumed that I have now ventured out of my house. And you are wrong. It is the third month and the tension has died away. I am extremely busy now, as I am juggling various activities at MUN Impact (which has truly changed my life) and studies. Seventeen hours a day isn't enough to complete my work.

I have no time to overthink and have formed a similar schedule to "normal life". I am finally content with my life!

With love,
A content Nikki.

Niharika D'Souza, 16, India

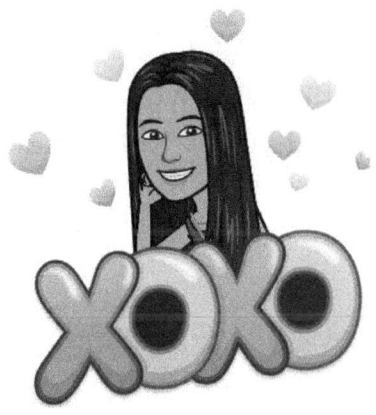

Make some Daily Affirmations

To get you started:

1. Today, I feel happy and motivated!
2. I feel strong and ready for a new day!
3. I am positive and confident!

Okay, now you create three!
(then create more!)

1. _____

2. _____

3. _____

When you wake up, take to the mirror and state your intent, make your case!

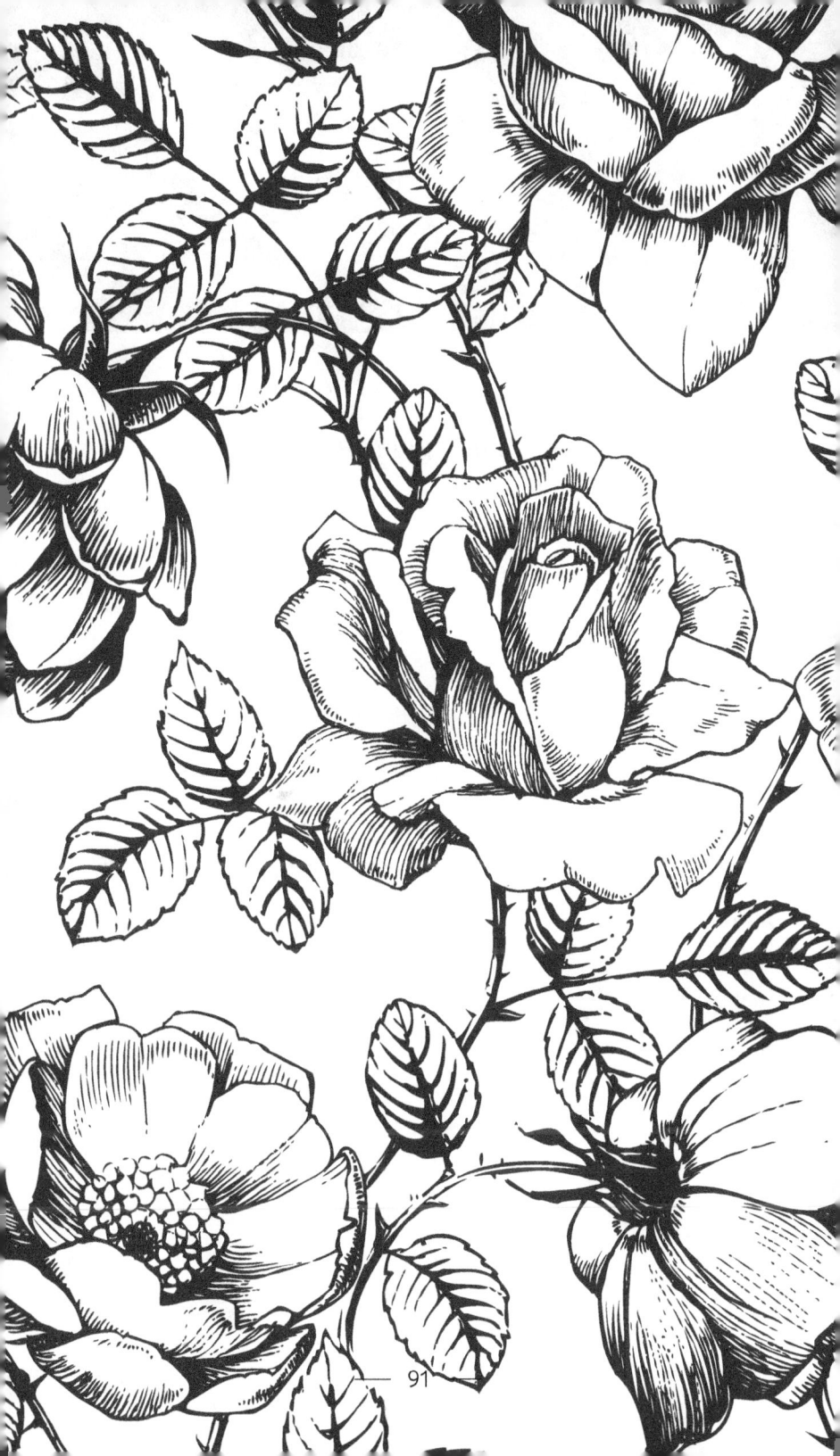

YEAR BOOK
STYLE

Screenshot class sessions on zoom, print and glue here.

PANDEMIC
Pre-Covid-19

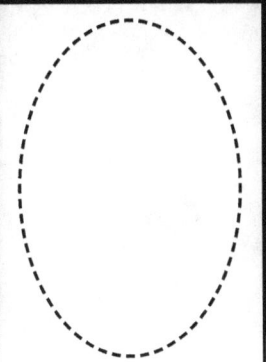

Print & paste favorite picture of yourself

YEAR BOOK STYLE

Pass around for friends to sign
(put on a mask and be careful!)

BACK TO NORMAL
Post-Covid-19

Print & paste picture of your face once your life is back to normal.

The Sun Always Rises

During lockdown we are forced to stay indoors and cut out meeting our friends, relatives and family members....but that doesn't stop us from having fun and spending time with our family and in fact we become closer.

The lockdown has given us a chance to go back to the days when family time was the most important time of the day...... every house becomes a worship place and our Almighty Lord protects us and makes us feel blessed and safe ..and I thank God for that...

In quarantine everyone is affected mentally and physically. We get anxious and devastated but still even if there are ups and downs we get to live together more and spend time more ...

I spent a lot of time with my family and communicated with my friends through online ways. Even if we were in quarantine ..I still learned a lot. I had participated in free online programs. I gained a lot of knowledge. The times I was bored and sad I gained more spiritually and I communicated with my friends and family...

During these hard times I know a lot of people are suffering like anything but I thank god for keeping me and my family safe and well. I didn't like not being able to see my relatives in my hometown and my beloved Grandma...

I miss those times usually we would go to India and see my Grandma and relatives .... but instead here we are stuck but at least we could still communicate and see them online.

I see this lockdown in a positive and happy way and none of us got sad and vexatious which affects our mental health... I am having a great time at home right now.

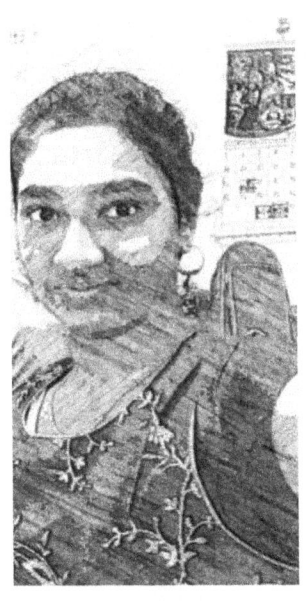

The realization that all the dramatic things that resulted from the virus and things we undertook to save ourselves and our planet have temporarily creating positives and that they really do seem to make a difference has lifted my spirits.

Whether it's the smog clearing over industrial cities during the shutdown, or the reduction of our daily lives to the simple basics, what we're experiencing now is a fast-forward into the way we must live in the future.

Everything is not locked down.

Love is not locked down.... Family time is not locked down.... Kindness is not locked down.... Creativity is not locked down.... Learning is not locked down.... Conversation is not locked down.... Imagining is not locked down.... Reading is not locked down.... Relationships are not locked down.... Praying is not locked down....Meditation is not locked down.... Work is not locked down....

The sunrise is not locked down....

Gladys Sophia, 12, India

No time to travel?

Color your mood while creating a story in your head of all the things you'd do if you could, in the location that contains these landmarks.

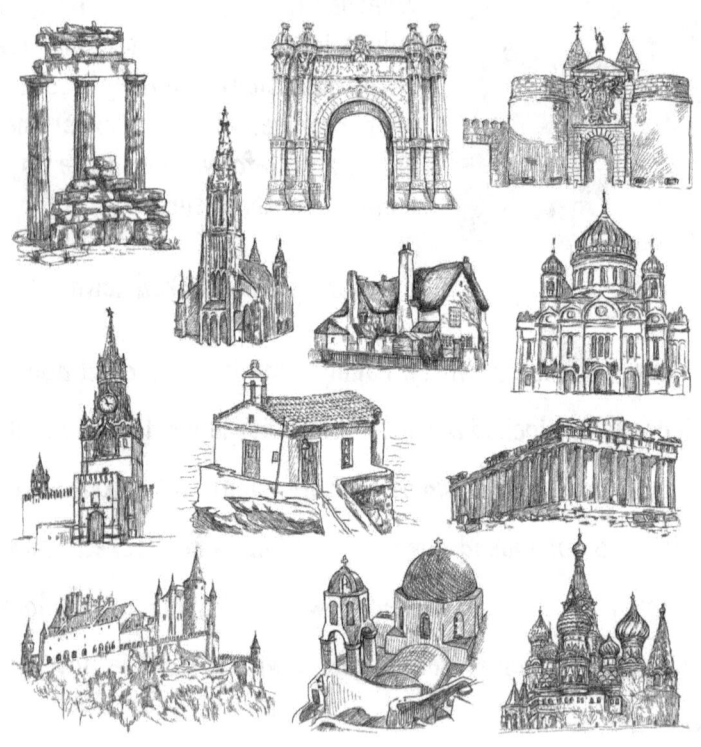

My travel wish list includes:

_____

_____

```
        CONFIDENCE
        O
        CONFIDENCE
        F
     CONFIDENCE
        D
   CONFIDENCE
        N
CONFIDENCE
        E
```

get it, got it, good!

Repeat Out Loud:

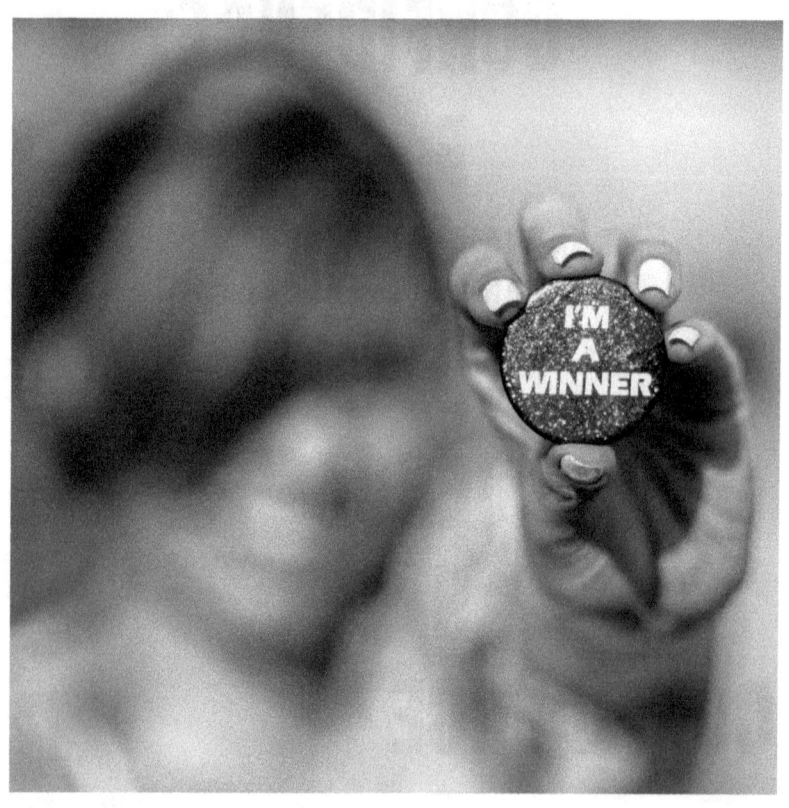

I will come out of this situation better than ever!

Can't get to the theatre?
Act out a scene from the Opera!

Set the scene, learn your script, and Action! Act out with a friend also in need of lockdown distraction. (If you recall this scene below from English Literature required reading, reward yourself later for your cultural sophistication) ☺

<u>Use this example, pretend you're Auditioning for role:</u>

A drawing-room in a Vienna hotel, richly appointed and newly furnished in the style of the 1860's. Adelaide is seated at a table, opposite the fortune-teller, Zdenka, in boy's clothes and seated at another table, busy with all kinds of papers (bills that have been piling up):

FORUNE-TELLER
The cards are more auspicious than they were last week.

ADELAIDE
I hope they are.
There is a knock at the door.
We cannot be disturbed.

ZDENKA
(answers the knock; somebody hands her a letter at the door)

ADELAIDE
(shaking her head)
Not now! Put it down there.

ZDENKA
At least it will have company!

ADELAIDE
Still, child. What do the cards say? Tell me! I'm so upset and worried I can't sleep at night.

...

Seek out the rest, it's superb!
Eternal thanks to Richard Strauss

The Comeback

Dear diary

I'm here again, this time I'm traumatized by the fact that everyone is dying because of the coronavirus. I'm scared that I might die. Being in Lesotho makes it worse because we don't even have enough resources to fight the virus. I ask myself every day, how are we going to fight the virus, the one thing that has turned our lives upside down, the one thing that cannot even been taken down by countries we thought were well developed.

I won't lie and try act like I am okay, no I am not, I am scared, scared for my life, scared for the lives around me, also scared for every life out there. Trust me, it's really hard for me to see all those people (on news, papers, media etc) breaking down, crying for their loved ones who were killed by the virus.

I can't even sleep at night, this whole thing is too much, all I think about day and night is "who is next? Is it me? Am I also going to be one of the victims? the victims of covid, one of the people corona is going to be proud it has killed?" this is just sad. Look at us now, sad, bored, depressed, how long are we going to live like this? We are stuck in our homes, nowhere to go, all we do every day is sit, nothing productive.

Parents have lost their jobs due to covid, they are stuck in houses with children, nothing to feed them. Now people are not only dying due to corona also due to hunger. Life has turned into something we have never thought of, we have got a lot on our plate. Online learning has become

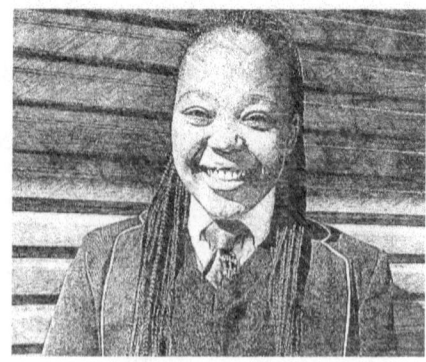

the only option for us as students even though it's really hard for us to get used to it. It really makes me sad that I am hopeless, but maybe there is still hope.

FAST FORWARD TO TODAY... I think we all have learnt a little bit about resilience in this time. Being isolated from the world has taught me a little about being strong. I think my nation is strong and we are going to fight no matter what. Even though we faced a lot of challenges during the lockdown I still tried to put myself together.

I took part in the SDG challenge to help me cope and make me feel like my voice matters. I also started investing more in my mental health as a student prioritising that spending time with my family has made me realise people need to care about their family because we will never know the last time we are going to see them.

It has also taught me that as people we have to take care of ourselves, do exercises, daily check-ups and all.

My writing has saved me from disappearing, the few poems and books I have written have given me hope not no give up. We are all prone to give up at this point in our lives but take it from a young girl who almost lost hope when she saw an unfamiliar certain of being isolated.

If I don't give up, what makes you think you should? A wise man once said the comeback is always stronger than the setback.

Moipone Selepe, 16, Lesotho

Today is _____

Dear Diary,

_____

_____

_____

_____

_____

_____

_____

_____

_____

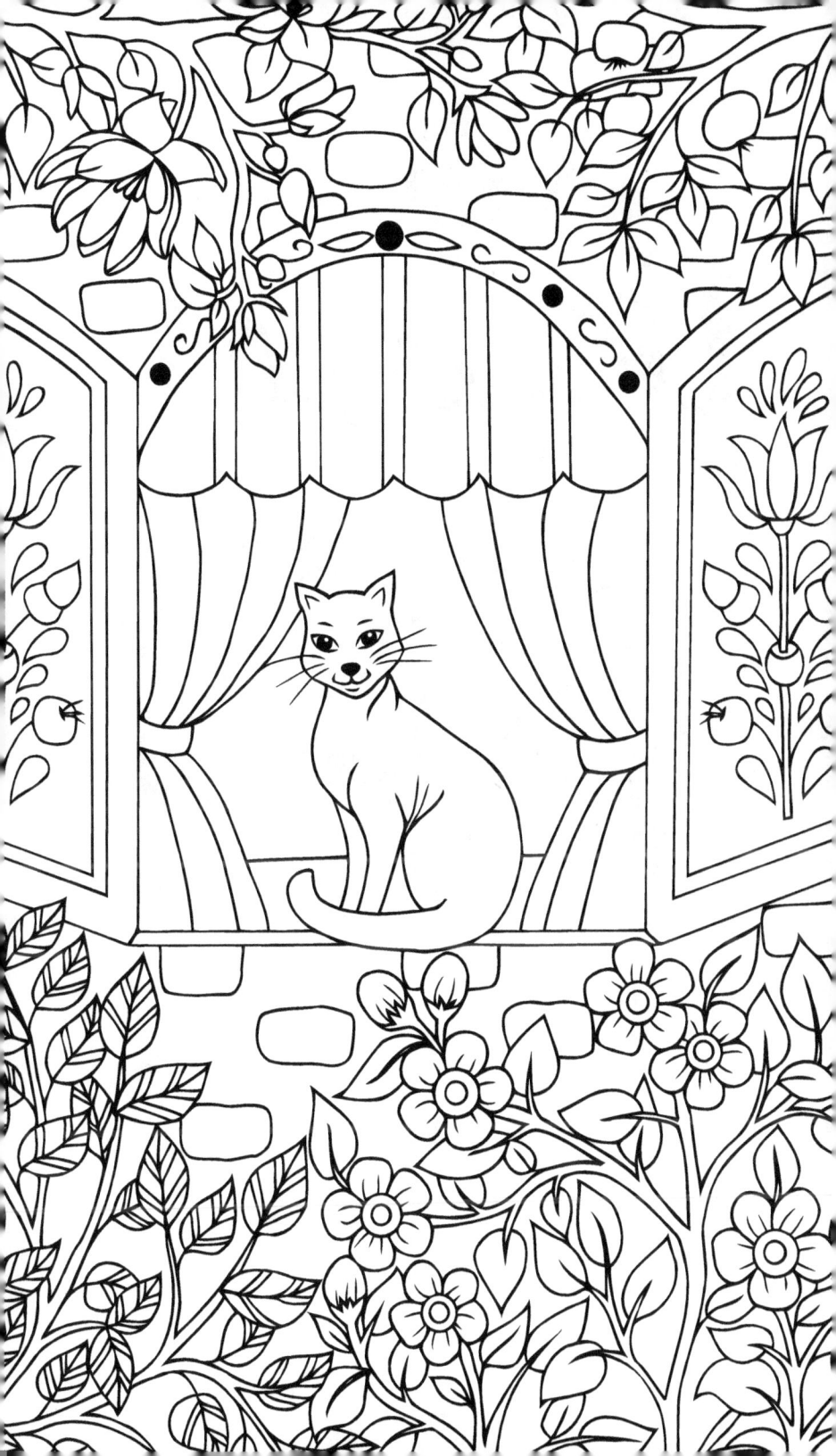

Dance!

Like there is no hidden camera recording your every hot move

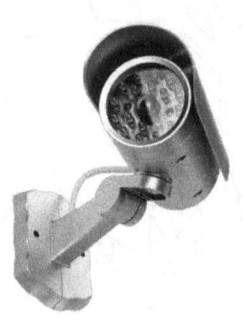

Word Dump

Add your one or two word descriptions relating to the things that have you stressed out about this horrible pandemic.

Counting Blessings

It's difficult to stay at home for five straight months. But I did - I stayed.

Ever since the COVID-19 pandemic wave hit my country, I had been uncertain, nervous and extremely sad. I couldn't visit my friends or relatives. All I did was attend online school once a day.

I was depressed.

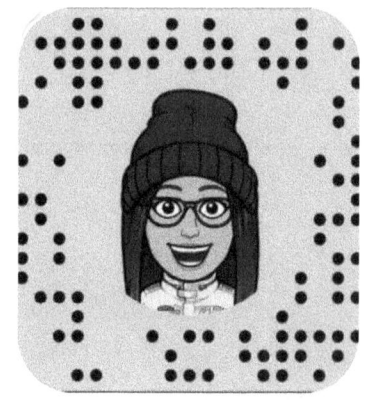

It's not human nature to be sad, but the very thought of not having something you really want but do not really need - that's human nature. That very behaviour had overtaken me and I sat down to ponder, to recollect my thoughts.

I looked over me, and there was a roof. I looked down and I had perfectly beautiful clothes draped over me. I had just come back from a lovely dinner my mother had cooked, and my father, my sister and I were settling down to play some type of game I didn't really like.

But did I like it? Did I actually be grateful for everything for everything I had? Millions of people are probably desolate , desperate and struggling for survival. Didn't I have enough?

That question eluded me. I finally decided- yes, I should be happy for what I have right now. I am happy. I'll always be happy for what I have, never sad for what I don't. Ever since I realized this simple philosophy, I've been learning to see the good in my life, which is actually a lot.

I've been pursuing my hobbies and volunteering for the good. I'm doing schoolwork, spending time with family and calling friends occasionally to catch up.

I'm happy now, and hopeful this wave of uncertainty passes soon. I hope everyone sees the blessing of what they have right now, and immediately have a smile on their faces.

Neha Varadharajan, 13, India

IDEA

GET

CREATIVE

Build something, do some crafting, cook! Bake some bread or a cake. Find or make some cookie cutters (who cares if it's not really a holiday, you deserve it–you're home and you make your own rules!) Make some festive, decorative and yummy cookies!

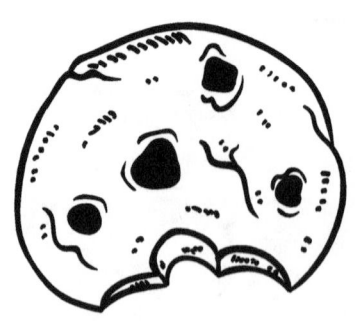

> *"The best way to find yourself is to lose yourself in the service of others."*
>
> Mahatma Gandhi

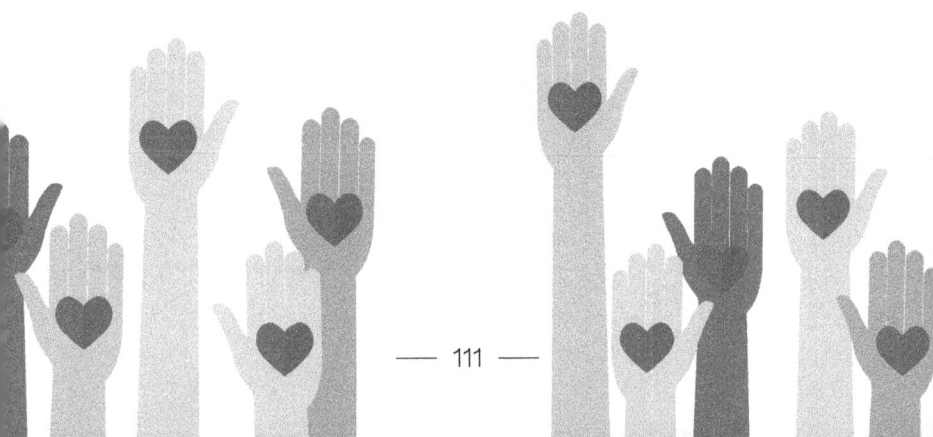

List 8 of your favorite comfort foods backwards:

Doritos = __SOTIROD__

___ = _____

___ = _____

___ = _____

___ = _____

___ = _____

___ = _____

___ = _____

Inhale

DO A BREATHING EXERCISE OF YOUR CHOICE

Exhale....Ahh...

Repeat...Lighten up

Upward & Onward

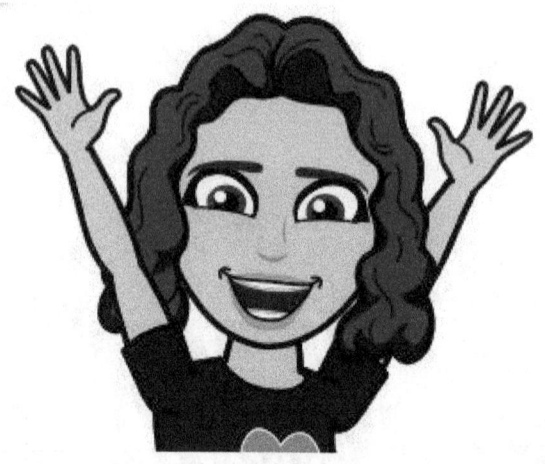

Upon hearing about the opportunity to contribute to this book I was sent into this state of visceral excitement that I often experience when a youth voice is uplifted. It dawned on me that I'd be able to emit a sort of signal to others: "did you feel that too?... tell me you felt that too."

I share my experience of a world that mankind let COVID steal, in hopes that it contributes to others' resilience, to feel comfort too amidst the difficulty.

I've kept a journal for the past year or so confiding in its pages with entries placed in a manner secret enough that I can write without my anxiety brain placing too much of a dam on my stream of consciousness. Yet the quantity of entries has barely shifted upward since the start of quarantine!

This surprises me as I feel a shift in my connection to journaling; it no longer involves condemning frustrations that take up too much headspace to paper and forgetting about them. Instead, I evolved a new approach to journaling as a result of the inevitable toll that COVID-19 has taken on the world that I so deeply love.

The work that I commit my free time to and will pursue as a career is a resource for humanity and gives me a reason to reconcile the anxiety brought on by COVID-19 instead of shoving it away to continue with my passions and not just survive.

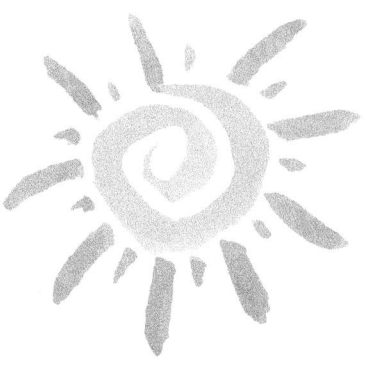

I made journaling into a teaspoon of sugar to choke down the chaos making me able to cope instead of settling and as side effects of the pandemic go; this new approach forced by the pandemic is pretty great in my mind.

Are some days harder to get through and process than others? Of course, but with my accepting mind, I get to visualize those fluctuations and be reminded that I am alive and am living instead of feeling overcome with hopelessness for the future.

So here's to strength in sugar in hopes that I can carry it with me as well as pass it on.

Sydney Rico, 17, USA (Cuban American)

I am grateful for

Today	Everyday	Most days

**Take a walk,
let nature work her magic.**

take it from Albert Einstein,

"Look deep into nature, and then you will understand everything better."

Mind over Mood

We cannot flip a switch on the emotions that affect us: anxiety, shame, embarrassment, anger, jealousy, sadness. But we can inhale a deep breath, step back and take a few moments to consider WHY we are feeling certain emotions at a given time. You have it within yourself to influence your own behavior. Isn't that awesome?!

Even if you are livid, you need not act with rage. You can decide to speak slowly and deliberately, or even smile, despite the volcanoes erupting in your head. These are just two tips – and practiced skills that will help you navigate the flood of feelings that flummox your life. You'd do really well to have your intellect, your logic, rule your decisions.

And, don't dwell on whether or not you've made the right decisions. If reason rules, you'll be more likely to make choices that'll hurt you less if you're wrong; and reward you more if you're right. Never allow emotions to be the boss of you.

Don't throw something when you're mad; don't give something away because of pity; don't reply when frustrated; and never go grocery shopping on an empty stomach! When sentiment rules behavior, the likelihood of regretting your actions is high.

Alternatively, when you approach all matters with practical impartiality, you will find greater peace with your circumstances. If a bully calls you an idiot, and you smile and walk away, they will be the worse for the interaction. When others throw their emotion at you, remember that you are not obliged to accept them or to respond in kind. It's THEIR problem.

> "Negativity is as destructive a disease as any virus. Unchecked, it will kill your spirit."
> Dad

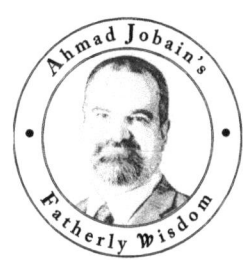

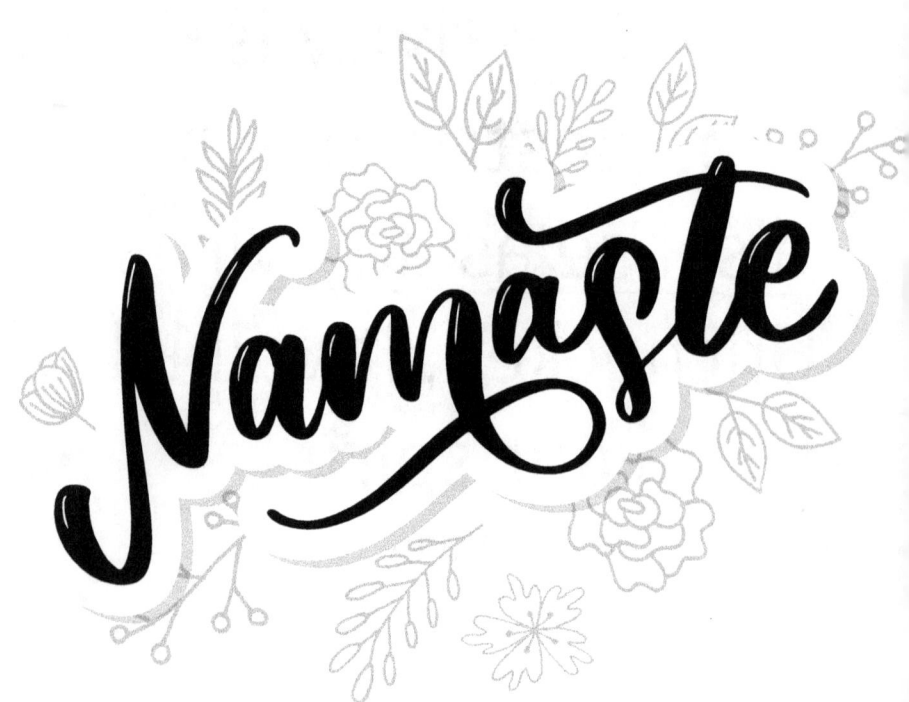

Feeling Bogged Down?

Not only will you feel lighter immediately and have better breath,

FLOSS!

(and then brush with great smelling toothpaste)

insert some teeth

flossing is good for your heart and studies suggest this can add years to your life.

(Google it!)

Maybe you'll even make some new friends, once the quarantines are all lifted for good!

(Your pleasant breath will make wearing a mask more pleasant, too!)

Have $5?!
You can become an Investor!
(Ask your parents first, please)

> APPS! for micro/fractional shares of publicly traded companies!

- **Charles Schwab Slices**

- **Robinhood**

- **Acorns**

- **Stash**

i.e. if a publicly traded stock like Apple (AAPL) has a price of $116.60 per share and you invest $3.50, you own about .03 or 3% of ONE share of that stock!

These fractional shares are available now to the public and popular with new or young investors who can try investing in the publicly traded stock market without large financial commitments or exposure- BUT stock investing IS STILL RISKY. ASK YOUR PARENTS first!

Choose your month + make some <u>short term goals</u>!

SAT						
FRI						
THU						
WED						
TUE						
MON						
SUN						

Consider How Realistic your Frustrations or Fears

about life returning to normal.

Current Outlook   *The Likely Outcome*

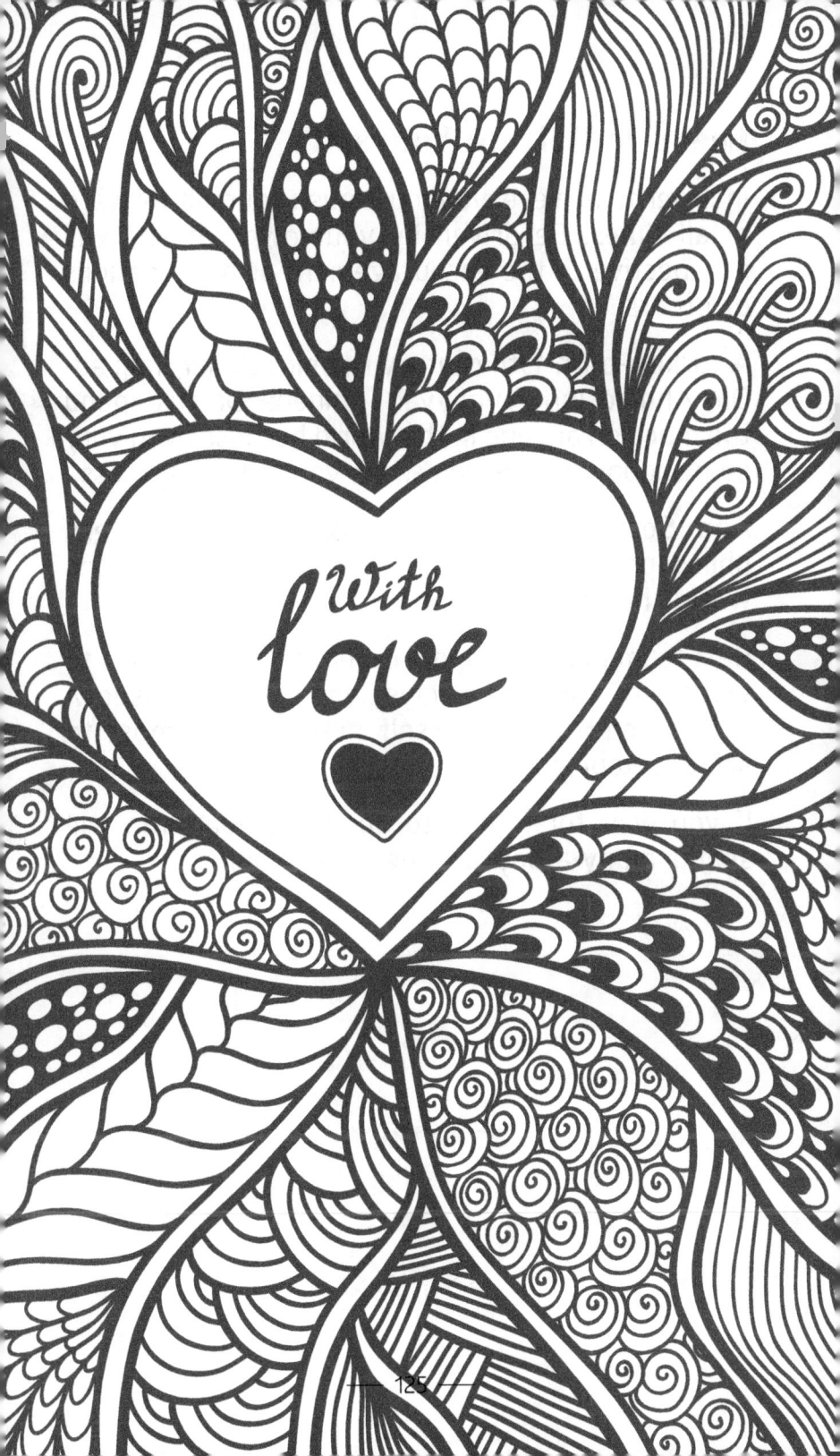

Learn to Rely on Yourself

In order to achieve, you must push yourself forward at all times. Be driven by your own wit and will irrespective of the encouragement or machinations of others.

A Turkish-born 13th century Islamic scholar, Taqî ad-Dîn Ahmad ibn Taymiyyah, opined: "Don't depend too much on anyone in this world because even your own shadow leaves you when you are in darkness."

And Socrates, the Greek founder of Western philosophy, admonished: "If a man would move the world, he must first move himself."

Be a team player, support others and allow them to work with you. But always keep expectations low; and depend upon yourself first and foremost to achieve your goals.

If you wait for others to open the door, you will spend many-a-day staring at a plank.

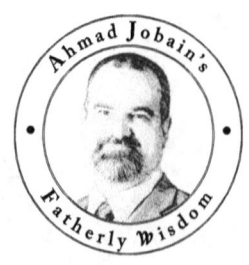

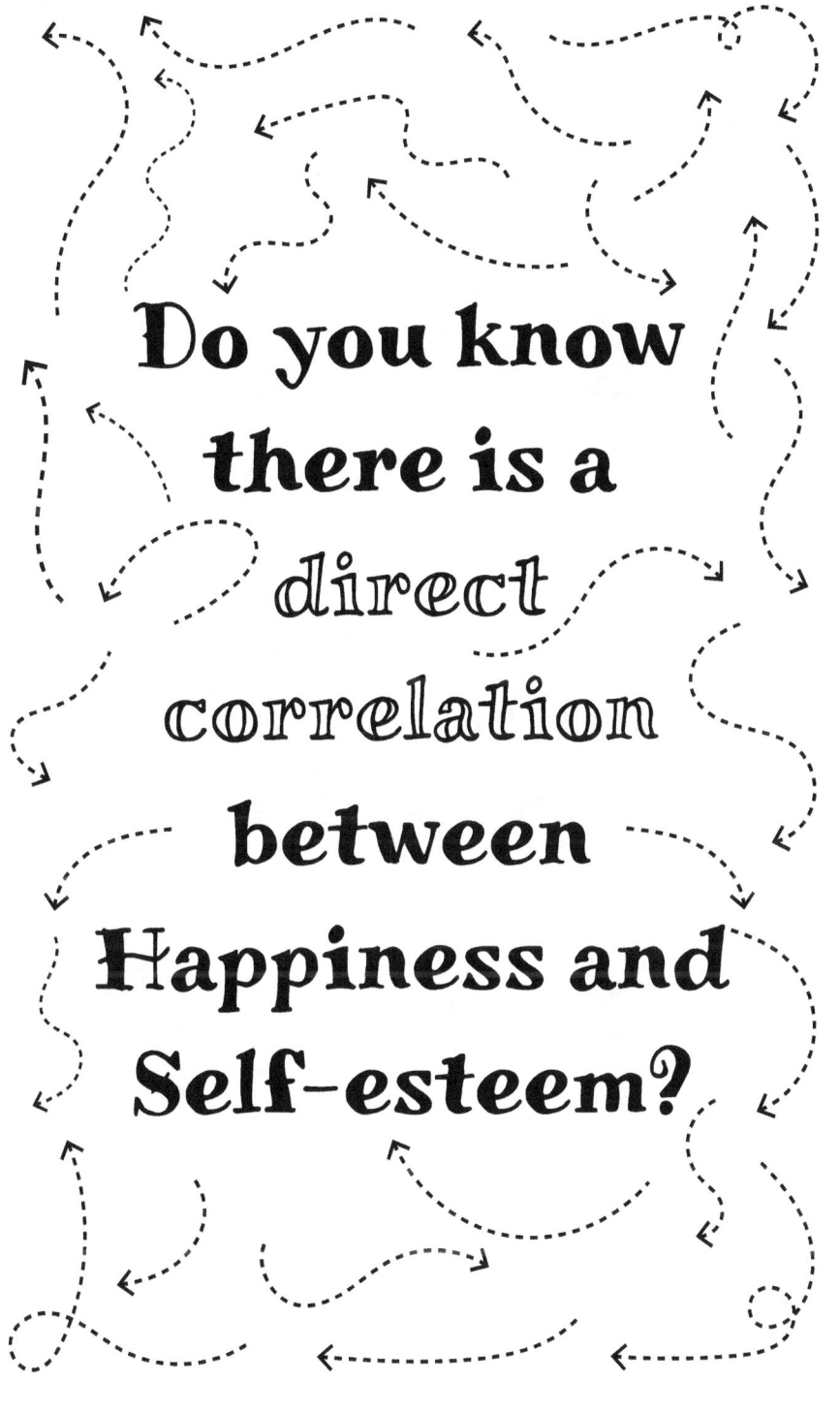

Confucius wisdom, modernized! to consider:

"The (wo)man who says (s)he can or the (wo)man who says (s)he can't are both correct."

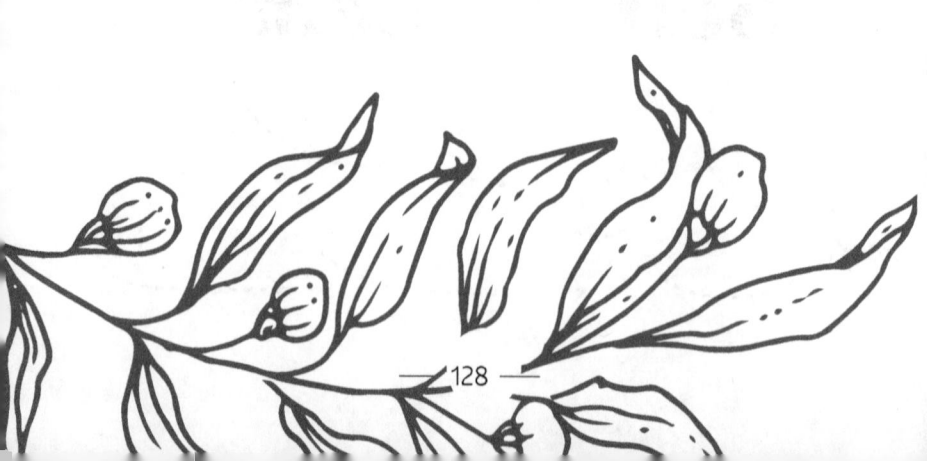

Put Future Possibilities in Focus

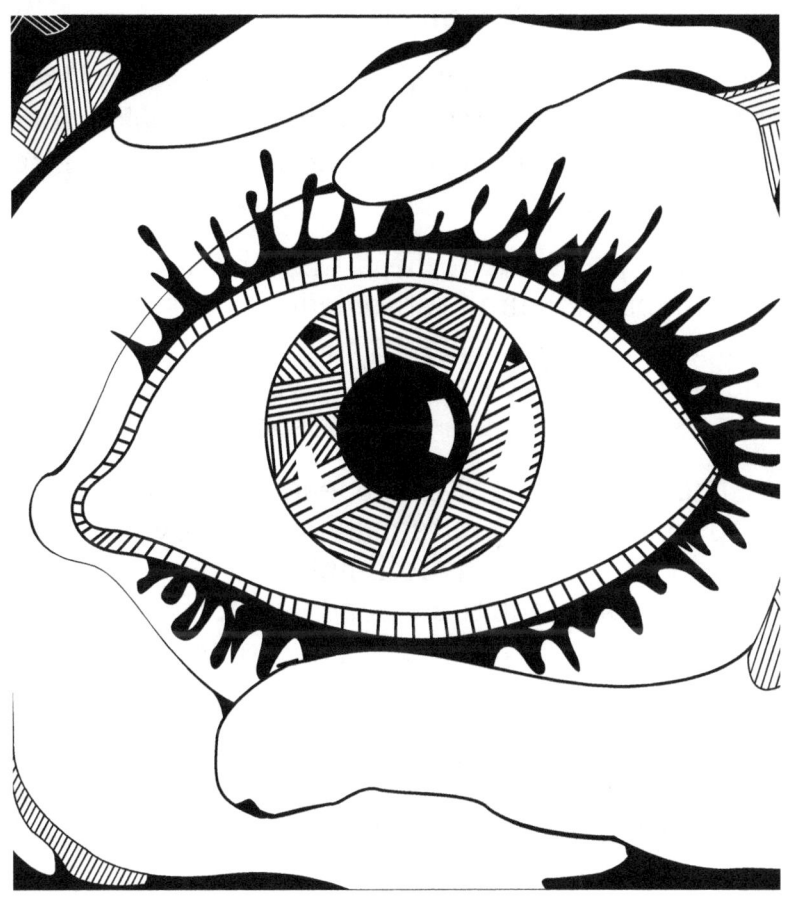

No matter how long Covid-19 lasts, life goes on, as good as YOU make it!

Hone your Personal Power & Fortify your Future

True personal power is not that which you wield over others, it is the ability to control yourself despite the comportment of others.

If you are able to master your mind, it is less likely that feelings and reactions will neither break before a boss or bully nor will you falter when trying to achieve anything.

Whether you want to be a CEO or will be happy flipping burgers until retirement, it doesn't matter as it's nearly impossible to change your character; and you need to be content in your own skin – as long as you know the consequences.

Just remember that being a leader or professional is optional; but if you remain unsure of your goals or how to go about accomplishing them, know unequivocally, indubitably and unambiguously that someone else or an intervening force will decide for you.

Your decisions are a reflection of your personal power. If you do not seek a position of leadership in life, that's okay, you can still focus on mastering and managing yourself!

And, if you do dream of leadership, you will need to master yourself as well master how to work and deal with others. In all cases, know that the strength to learn and persevere is within you; and not in what others determine for you. Only when you get that through your head will you have personal power.

If you are feeling down, discouraged, uncertain, **you are NOT alone!**

Remember,
"THIS TOO SHALL PASS"

Persian proverb

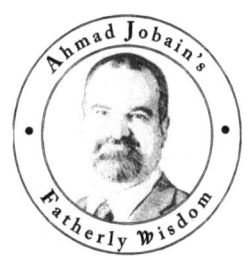

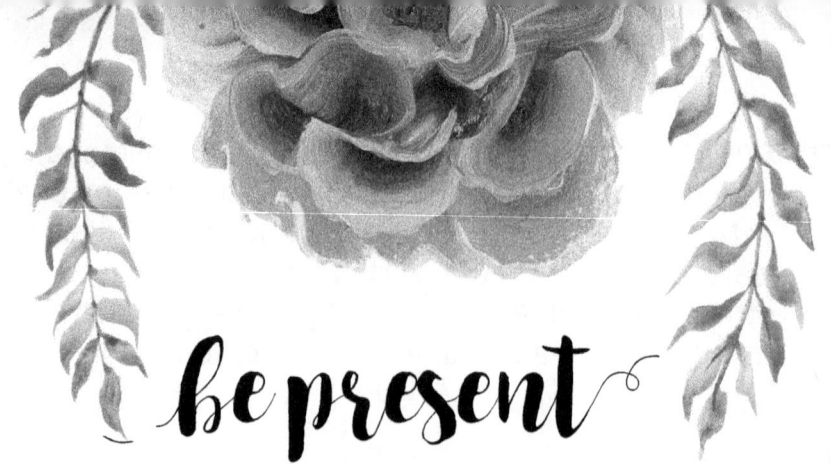

be present

Be here

Be now

Pay attention

Concentrate

The past is gone

The future hasn't arrived yet

Make today count

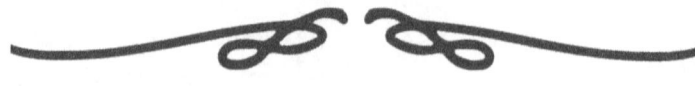

Exercise Much?

No nagging.

No judgments.

just ...consider it

it's proven to be uplifting to the spirit (not to mention your hiney)

Failure is a Word not a Sentence

When things don't quite go the way you plan, spend a few moments understanding the possible causes (preparation, circumstances, unforeseen factors); but never let the experience linger in your mind.

Overthinking will cause you to question your competence and skill. Americans define unsuccessful events as "learning experiences" for a reason – they represent an opportunity to see the matter you have just undertaken from a different angle.

Thomas Edison, the man who invented the lightbulb, alkaline batteries and much more, is reported to have said: "I have not failed. I have just found 10,000 ways that don't work."

And Winston Churchill, who led the British during World War II, rightly declared: "Success is stumbling from failure to failure with no loss of enthusiasm."

So, whether you have done poorly on an exam, received a bad review or fallen short of your goals, always analyze what your actions had been before you failed.

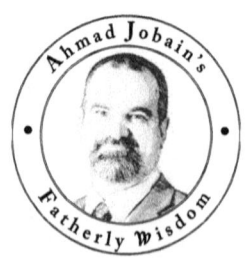

Consider your actions and how you conducted yourself. Plan better next time. Never dwell longer than necessary on the incident itself. Succeed wildly next time.

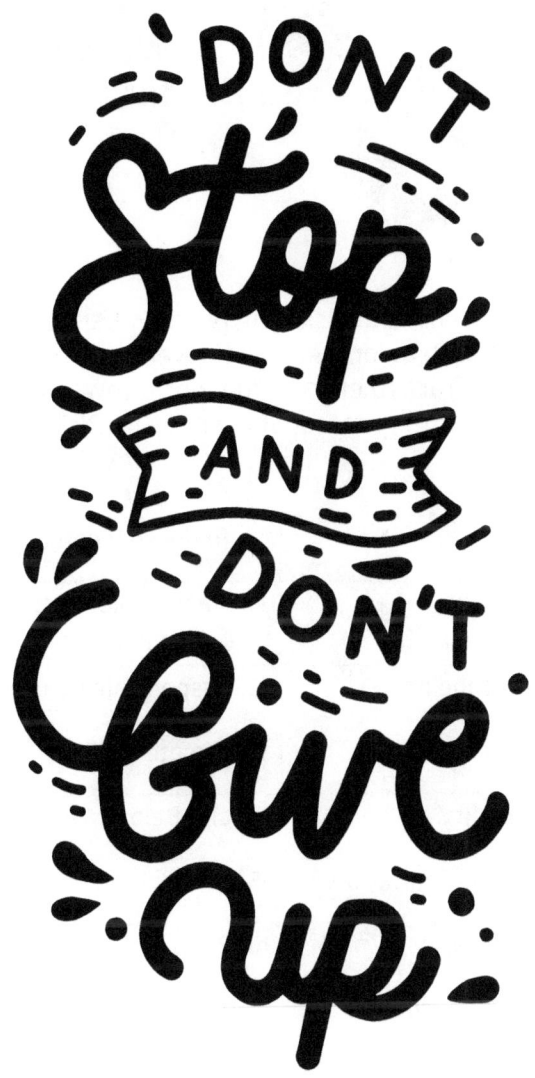

Advocating for SDG #3

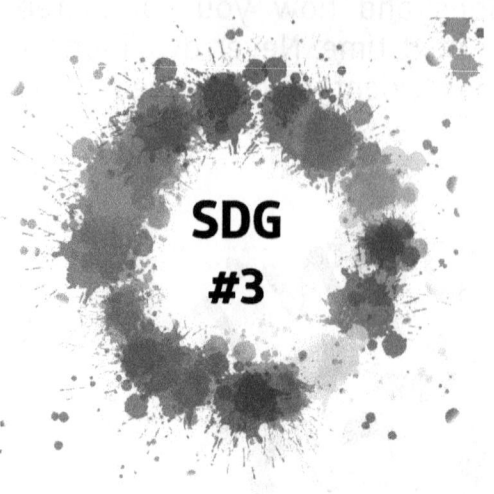

SDG #3 — Health & Wellbeing for all by 2030

In 2015 by consensus decision of 193 member states, the 17 UN Sustainable Development Goals were born. The "Global Goals" are an effort to engage the world toward resolution of Earth's greatest challenges by 2030.

1. No Poverty	10. Reduced Inequalities
2. No Hunger	11. Sustainable Cities & Communities
3. Health & Wellbeing	12. Responsible Consumption
4. Quality Education	13. Climate Action
5. Gender Equality	14. Life Below Water
6. Clean Water & Sanitation	15. Life on Land
7. Renewable Energy	16. Peace & Justice
8. Good Jobs & Economic Growth	17. Partnerships for the Goals
9. Innovation & Infrastructure	https://sdgs.un.org

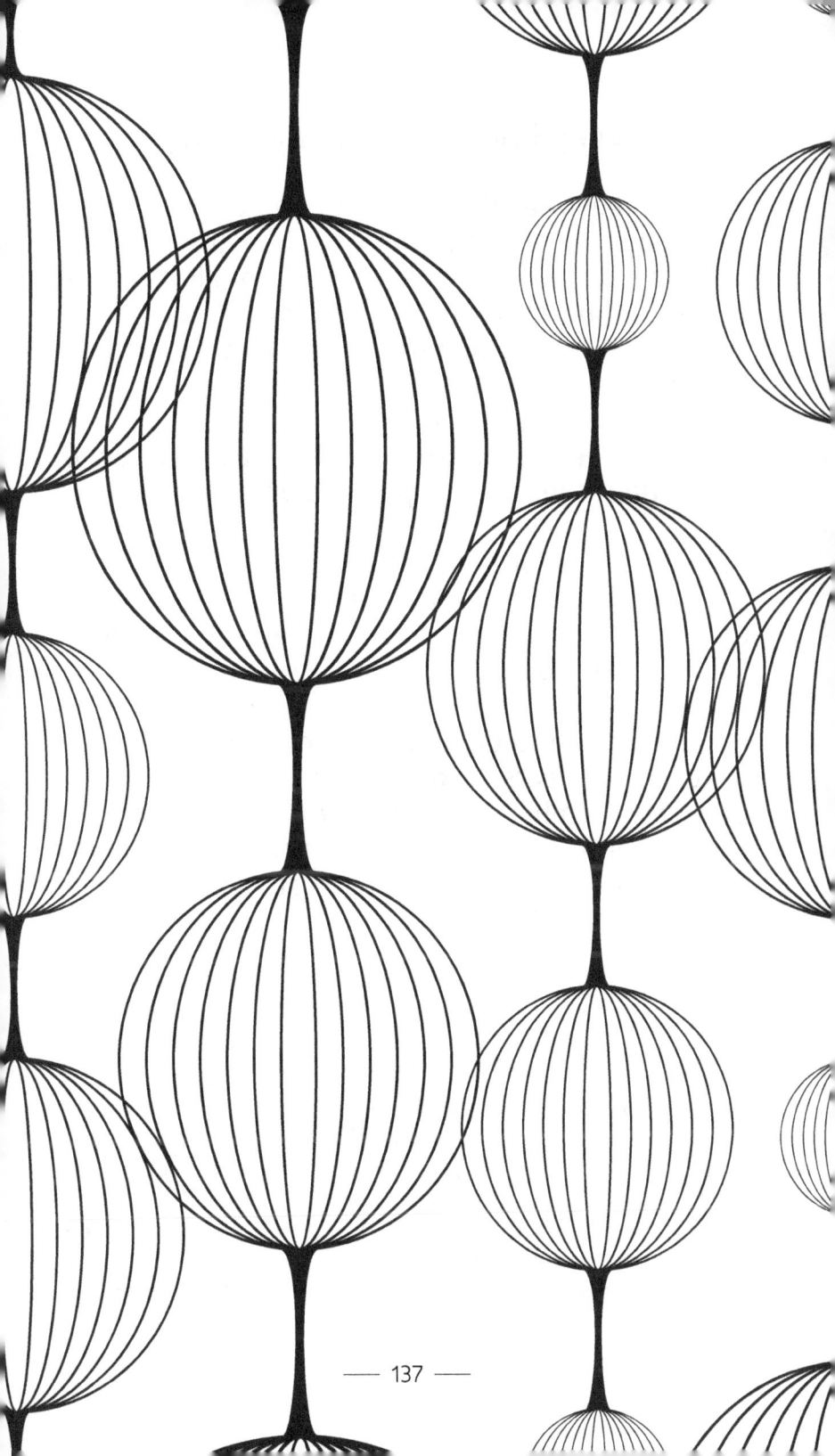

Furry Companions (aka Pets)

If you're feeling a bit 'incomplete' and you otherwise have positive relationships with humans (and the aliens among us), yet have no outlet for all your love and attention or your home is just too quiet, you might VERY carefully consider adopting a/n (rescue ☺) animal as a pet.

(Notice it doesn't say "if you're feeling bored" or "if you're prone to impetuous decisions")

And, if you're not quite sure and want to give pet parenthood a try without any negative effects on the "little guy", consider "fostering" an animal SHORT term. ☺

If you can plan to COMMIT part of your life for the next 10 - 20 years (God willing as long as possible) to a new member of the family (who won't argue, and is a great listener) you will find this is likely a fantastic decision and long term attitude enhancer and responsibility.

A PLEA: ...As LOVELY as pets can be for your wellbeing and positivity, they are A TON OF WORK and require actual (sometimes, near constant) attention. Especially "puppy-cats" and large parrots... So be sure you can commit because they deserve to be happy too. ♥

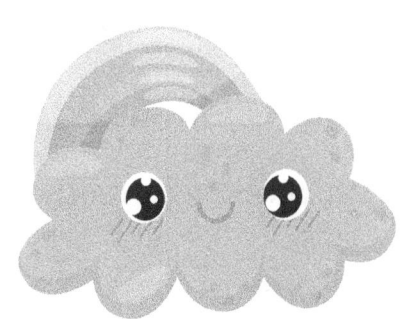

Be the rainbow and the end of someone's rainstorm

About the Panedmic & future...

I am healthy currently
YES_____   NO_____
*If NO, please call or see a doctor

What is/are the biggest issue(s) on your mind for the near future? (30-90 days)

_____

What is/are the biggest issue(s) on your mind for the mid-term future? (4-9 months)

_____

_____

Consider the things you can do or have done to address these issues

_____

_____

Meantime
____ I plan to social distance, wear a mask and be careful.
____ I plan to stay home & hope the outcome is positive!
____ I've given up all hope!
____ I am going about my life as normal as possible.

be kind
be nice

be gracious

give others a break, cut them some slack, look the other way

live & let live

Dissect!

Introspect!

Take stock
-(What are you all about?)

Express yourself

Buy a simple notebook + decorate it!

Then keep the creativity going

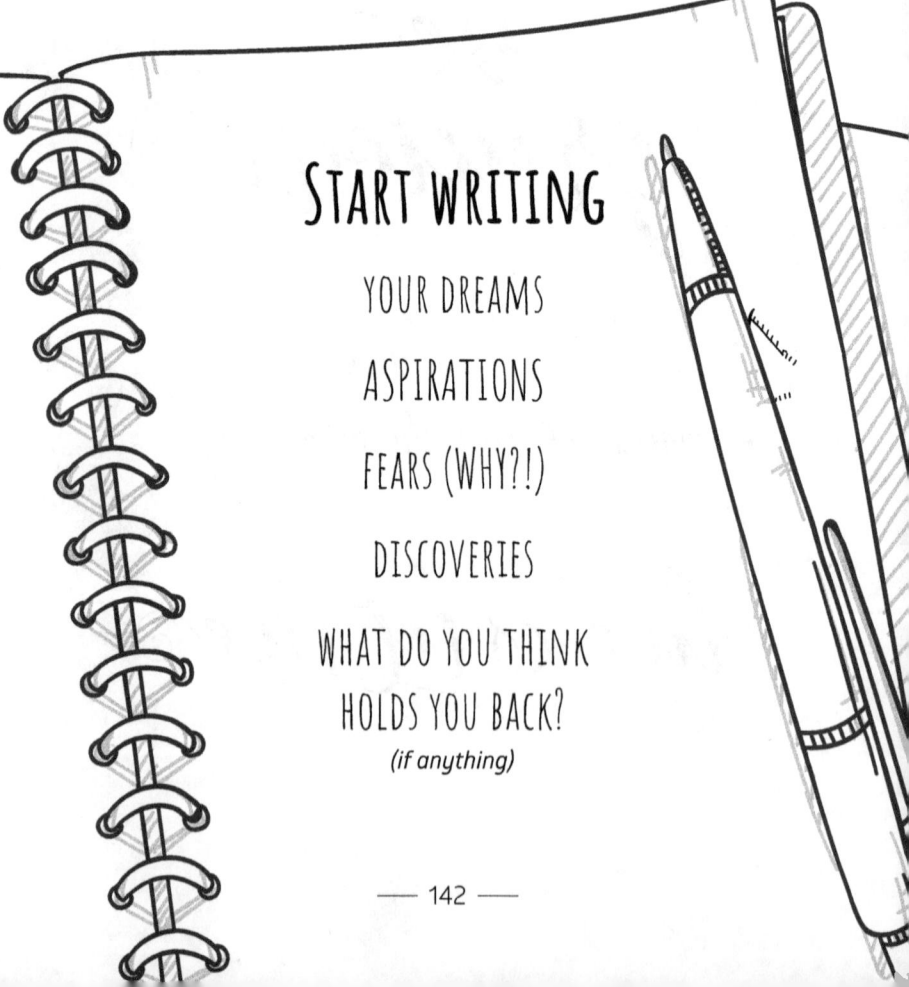

Start writing

YOUR DREAMS

ASPIRATIONS

FEARS (WHY?!)

DISCOVERIES

WHAT DO YOU THINK HOLDS YOU BACK?
(if anything)

You're only as Dumb as You Believe

Have you ever felt (or someone tried to make you feel) incompetent, incapable or idiotic? Life will put you in situations that make you feel that way; but just remember that if you can't get something done, it's only because you may not have had the training or experience to do it. If a colleague, teacher or friend – or even a parent - criticizes you or gives you negative feedback, it doesn't lower your worth. And don't take it personally the way in which the person has expressed his or her judgment of you.

Rather than say you need more training or guide you to a more appropriate course, if they articulate their words or behavior in a way designed to make you think they are superior, or you inferior, then the problem lies with them.

Never accept as true that something is wrong with you; only that, if you feel out of your depth, you're simply the right person in the wrong place or position. Believe in yourself because others will often only see in you what reflects their own judgment, not your potential.

Believe you can do anything because throughout your entire life, there will be plenty of people who may, perhaps unintentionally make you think otherwise and doubt yourself. Have your own back in this regard.

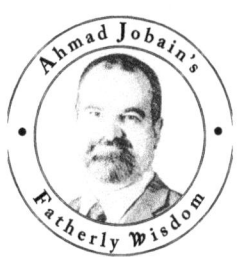

OMG
I AM SO
CUTE

Celebrate the Magical Healing Powers of...

*"There is nothing better than a friend, unless it is a friend with **chocolate**."* ~ **Linda Grayson**

*"Without pain, how could we know joy?' This is an old argument in the field of thinking about suffering and its stupidity and lack of sophistication could be plumbed for centuries, but suffice it to say that the existence of broccoli does not, in any way, affect the taste of **chocolate**."* ~ **John Green, The Fault in Our Stars**

*"Strength is the capacity to break a **Hershey** bar into four pieces with your bare hands - and then eat just one of the pieces."* ~ **Judith Viorst, Love & Guilt & The Meaning Of Life, Etc**

Viva La France! *"He showed the words "**chocolate cake**" to a group of Americans and recorded their word associations. "Guilt" was the top response. If that strikes you as unexceptional, consider the response of French eaters to the same prompt: "celebration."*~ **Michael Pollan, In Defense of Food: An Eater's Manifesto**

*"All you need is love. But a little **chocolate** now and then doesn't hurt."* ~ **Charles M. Schulz**

Selfish Sensibility

You will rarely meet a person who loves anyone or anything more than they love themselves. Whether or not they admit it – or even blatantly know it – it is a different matter... Most people put self-interest and self-preservation high on their list at the expense of even their closest and dearest friends and family.

Sure, there are exceptions; but you won't have the luxury of learning who these people are before you're hurt or disappointed. Don't fight it; and don't despair. This doesn't mean that most people are evil or malicious (though some certainly are). It just means that most are not going to put your interests ahead of theirs. And neither should you put your interests behind those of others!

But, to be certain, you should be considerate of others. Give someone in need a hand, help out when you can and when it's not at great sacrifice to you or your needs or demands of your life. Just don't let others take advantage of you. This is where some healthy selfishness comes in really handy.

While there are those who deserve your attention, everyone should know that your time, your feelings, and your money are precious commodities. Don't give them away lightly. There are limits. Set them! And know that it's not unusual in life to find that once you've done someone a favor, few people seem to remember it; and fewer still will reciprocate.

Not because they're bad people; but because they've either put themselves first or yes, they take you for granted. Don't let this be your fault, your downfall, or a situation that gets you down. When it comes to priorities, you're numero uno (#1!).

Remember that.

Please.

We are all more the SAME than we are different.
#Humans

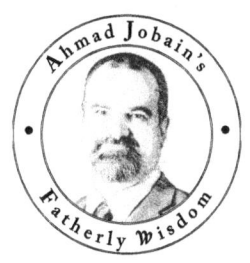

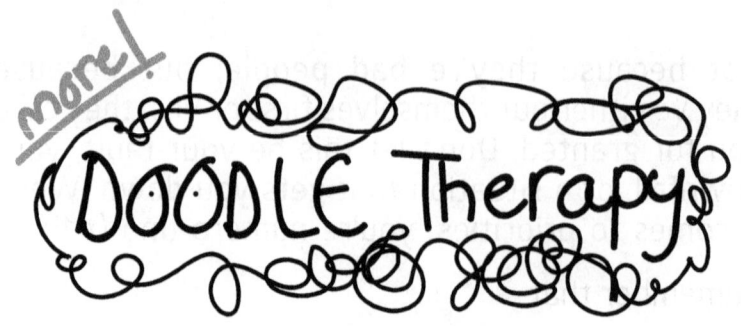

Draw your dream vacation

On Self Discipline:

Consider it a muscle that you need to work out, use, and practice strengthening it by setting small goals. Once you meet these, make some bigger ones. Quarantines are a great time to exercise and flex your discipline muscles.

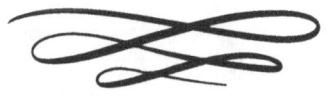

Commit, focus, be consistent and you'll go far!

SOMETIMES WE JUST NEED A LITTLE ATTITUDE ADJUSTMENT TO PUT THINGS INTO PERSPECTIVE

A little **tweak** here, and there..

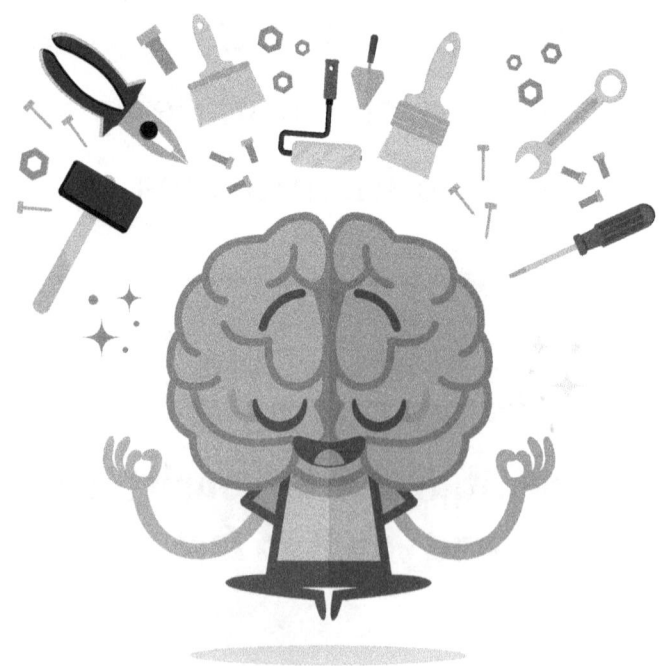

Doodle your plans for Winter

Ready, Aim, Shoot!

To succeed at hitting a target, clarity must be present. In life, you won't always know what you want – no one ever does; but you must still have objectives and targets, big or small.

Define your goal and then consider the steps needed to succeed. Whether a degree, a new job or your next holiday, "failing to plan, is planning to fail," a common management axiom attributed to Benjamin Franklin, one of the United States' Founding Fathers.

It's fun to live for the moment and be spontaneous, sure; but if you don't work with plans, you will find yourself increasingly aimless in life. That may be manageable when you're a young whippersnapper; yet as the years roll by, you will feel increasingly frustrated with your achievements, or lack thereof.

Never believe that a matter is too small to define a specific result you want to attain. Practice imagining the smallest but specific result you want to achieve, then strategize how to attain it.

As the years go by, you will find yourself enjoying the satisfaction of knowing where you are going and roughly how to get there.

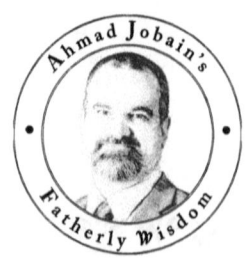

Consider your happiness not your unhappiness!

• • • • • • • • •

Practice positivity.
Every. Single. Day.

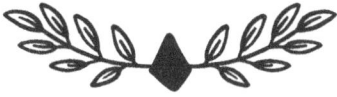

More, long-term AFFIRMATIONS

(Hint: You need to believe or want to believe these things)

I AM GOING TO GET ACCEPTED TO (..................................) UNIVERSITY IN 2022.

YOUR PARENTS...

If you're able, talk to them about how you're feeling and how you're processing, handling Covid-19. Share your thoughts and listen to theirs – ASK how THEY are doing.

And, go easy on your parents – they are human too (I know! Right?!) and sometimes even though they are the adult, adults need love and care too and it's hard to always be the strong one. Nurture them a bit right now.

As teenagers... sometimes, well... you know.

Just give them a hug and let them know that together, this Covid19 thing, as a family, "we got this!"

Celebrate Publicly, Complain Alone

Ella Wheeler Wilcox may not have imagined that a single line from a poem published in 1883 would be her most memorable legacy. *Solitude* begins with the stanza: "Laugh, and the world laughs with you; Weep, and you weep alone." The lesser known remainder explains: "For the sad old earth must borrow its mirth, But has trouble enough of its own."

Everyone has problems. Keep yours to yourself unless it is specific; and those to whom you speak have a solution they may be willing to provide.

Under no circumstances be the person who is always complaining.

Negativity is as destructive a disease as any virus. Unchecked, it will kill your spirit and doom you to a lonely, probably impoverished existence. And, you won't likely get invited to many parties.

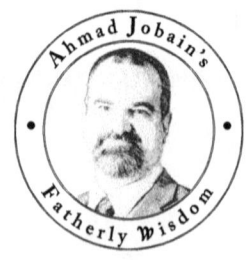

Get your coloring groove on

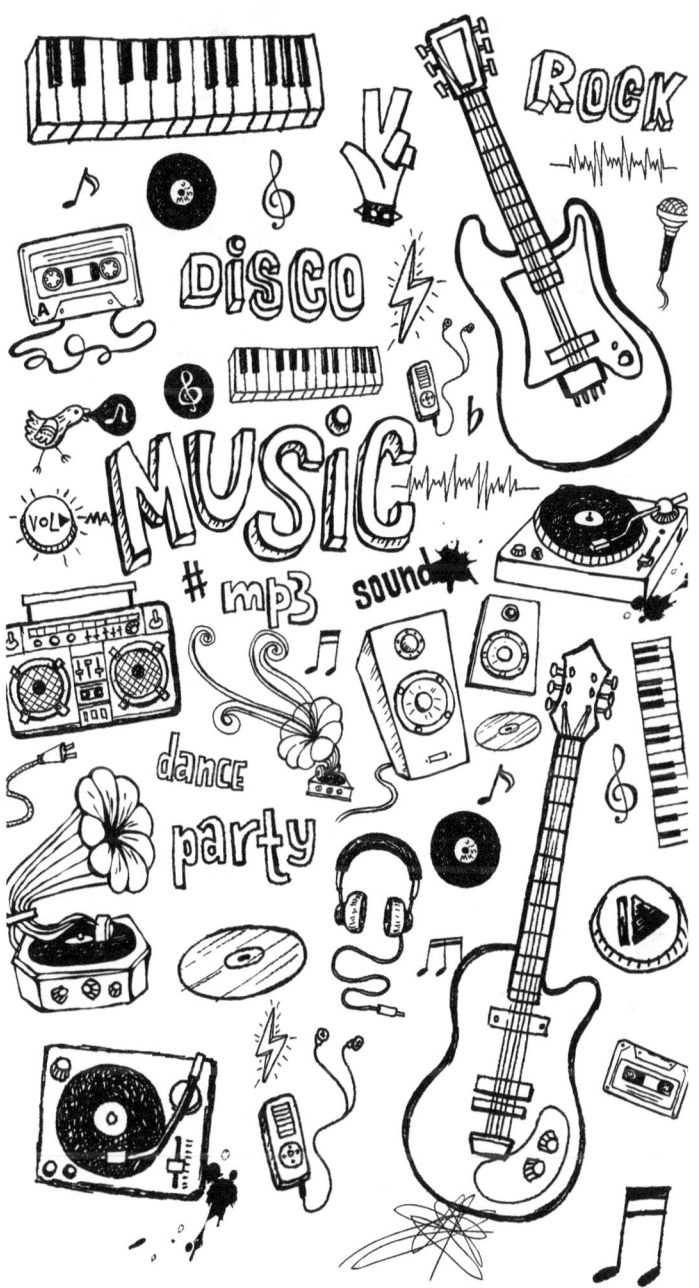

And... when all else fails in your efforts staring at 4 walls & a ceiling....

REMEMBER!

There is always delivery, online shopping & ice cream

Remind yourself of your favorite shops

_____
_____
_____
_____
_____

& favorite flavors

_____
_____
_____
_____
_____

Take Notice of the

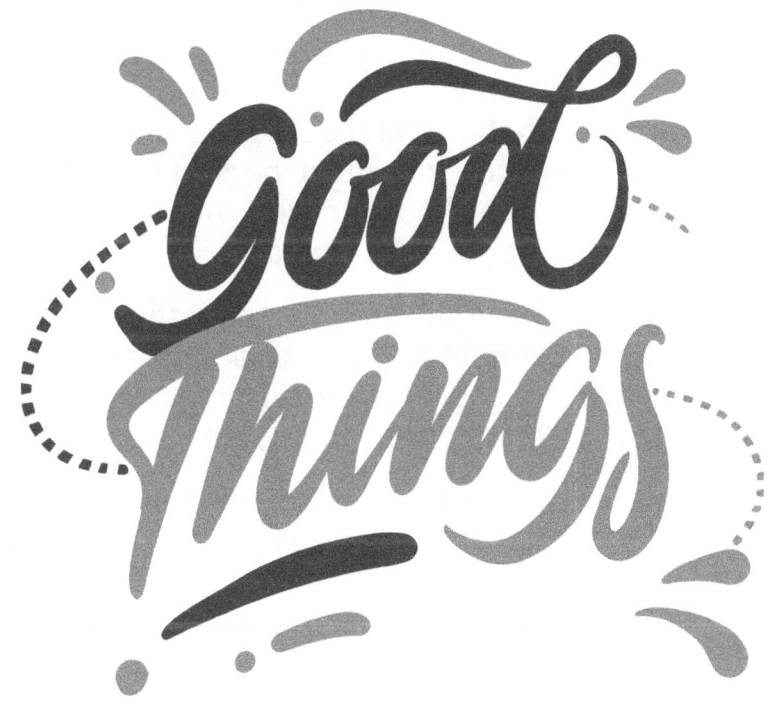

Choose a Great Mentor

No one is born experienced, even if they're born talented. You need a guide with some expertise to help you stay in charge of your life as much as you need one to help you navigate the working world.

Ideally, it'll be someone who is upbeat, accessible and open, one with whom you can talk candidly about your chosen life and career paths – or mull over the many options.

Whether you want to be an artist, a baker, a trader, a doctor or anything else, those who've walked that trail before you can help enlighten you.

If you're not sure who to reach out to, approach organizations specifically formed to foment mentorship for advice such as the International Mentoring Association and the European Mentoring & Coaching Council. You might be surprised how many of these will be happy to work with teenagers and young adults just starting out.

Also, seek out organizations that specifically focus on youth mentorship – their mentors are often millennials and provide closer generational assitance, understanding, input, and advisory.

If no one you know enthralls you with their wisdom, choose someone who has a blog or has written books and pore over their words. Their experience will not be yours and they won't give you input for your circumstances, yet hearing their perspective will certainly be better than clamoring through your own career blindly.

You can choose what advice to follow or ignore; but always take note of it, especially from those willing to share the knowledge and skills they've gained through their own challenges. It won't stop you from making your own mistakes; but at least you'll be better prepared to deal with them.

Take the time to listen to others, whether you think you already know what they mean or believe their opinions are baseless. Try to demonstrate modesty and absorb what others have to say.

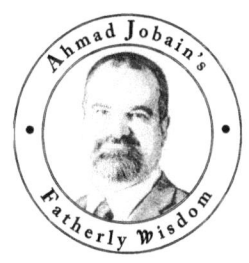

Share your homeland!

We'd love to learn more and hear about your country – Send a picture of this page to our email below or @mention us on social media and post! Now, tell us more about your homeland:

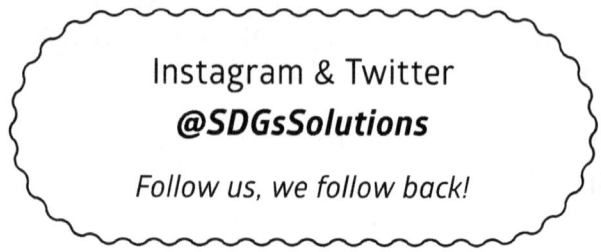

Instagram & Twitter
@SDGsSolutions

Follow us, we follow back!

1. Draw your nation's Flag:

2. Color your flag (coloring therapy works wonders!)
3. In which time zone are you located? _____
4. What's the population of your nation? _____
5. What's your nation's Capital? _____
6. What is your national animal or mascot?
   _____
7. Your favorite thing about home? _____
   _____
8. What is your nation most known for? _____
   _____

Treasure Map it!

The Toys & Goodies I Deserve!

A new bike? moped? car?

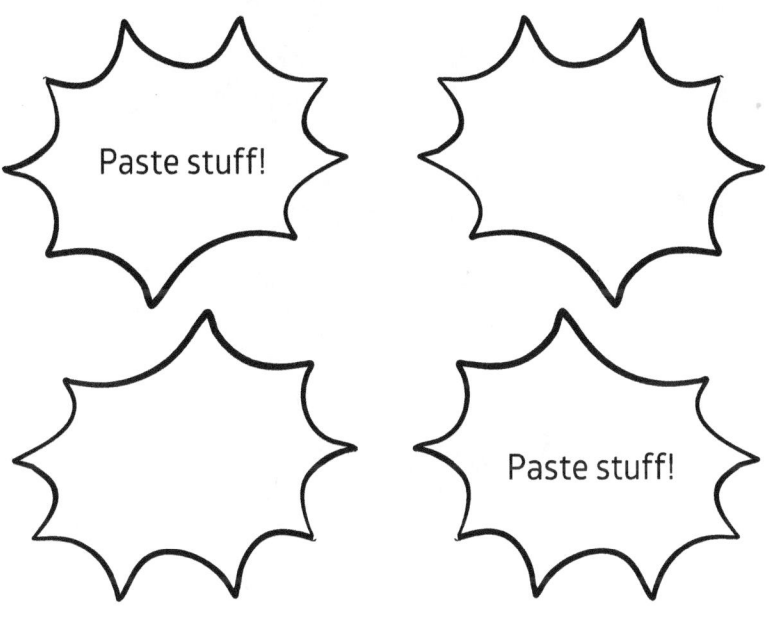

How about pasting a pic of yourself in the driver's seat?! You getting the hang of this? Great!

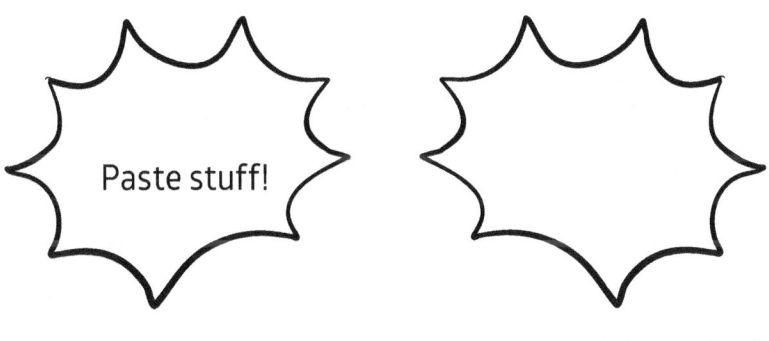

What else?!

"Teamwork makes the Dream work"

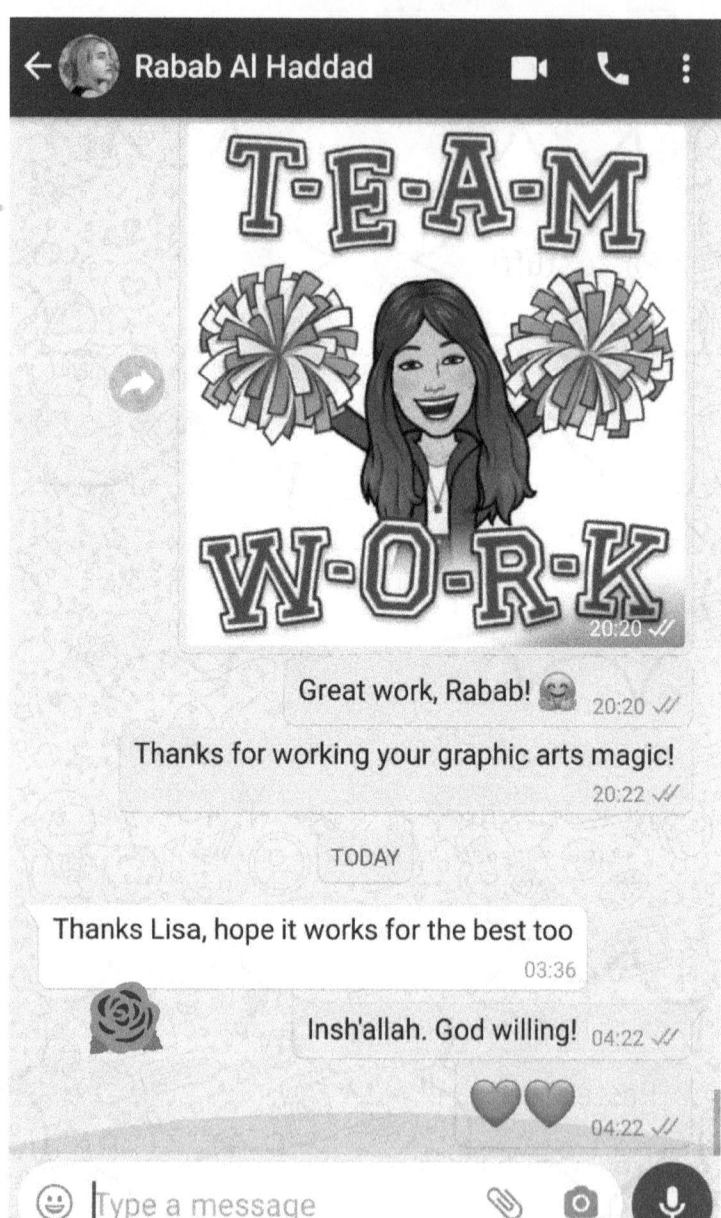

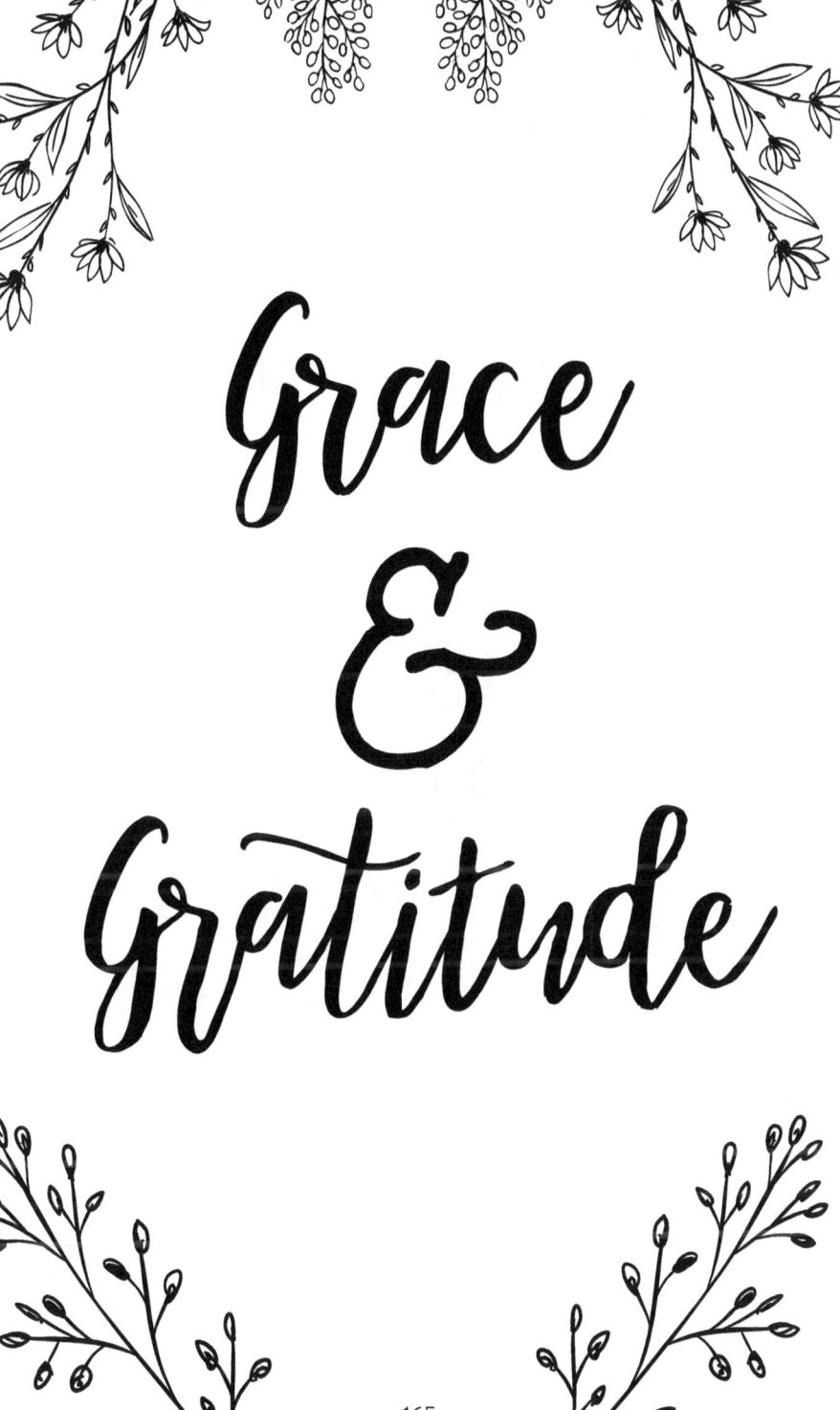

> "How far that little candle throws his beams! So shines a good deed in a weary world"
>
> William Shakespeare

Neither a Servant nor a Stalker Be!

There is no such thing as a one-way relationship because when it is, that means it's either servitude or stalking. And you don't want to be classified as either.

Put in mind that people may not stay in touch for a myriad of reasons. You could be irrelevant to them or they're overwhelmed with their day-to-day lives.

Whatever it may be, it simply means that you're not on the priority list. So, if someone doesn't return a call or attempt one in the first place, do not judge. They have their reasons, good or bad. Just like you have yours.

Reach out when you feel the urge to connect but don't over do it and learn to let go if you're being ghosted.

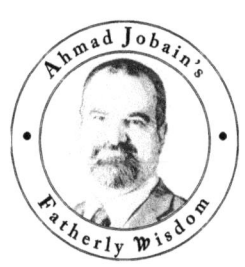

Mindful Eating

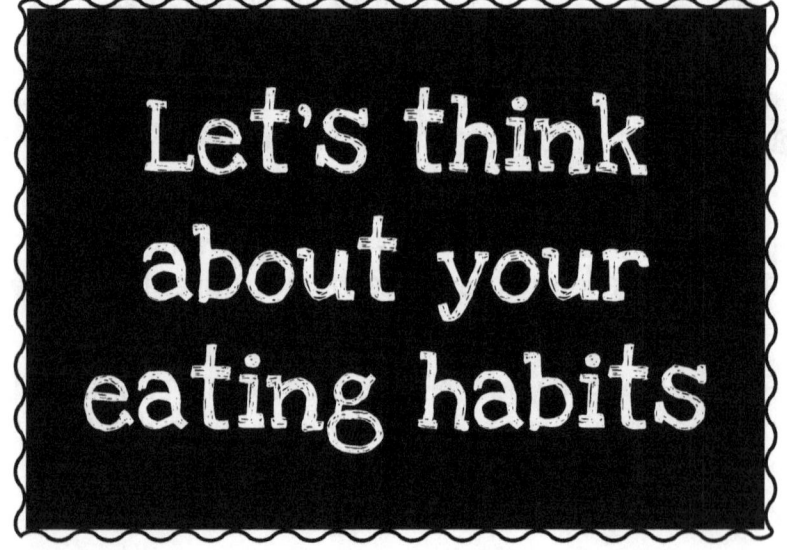

What good habits do you already have that you can build on?

What do you want to change?

What can you do to make that change today?

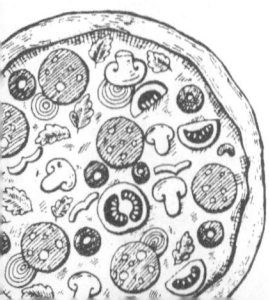

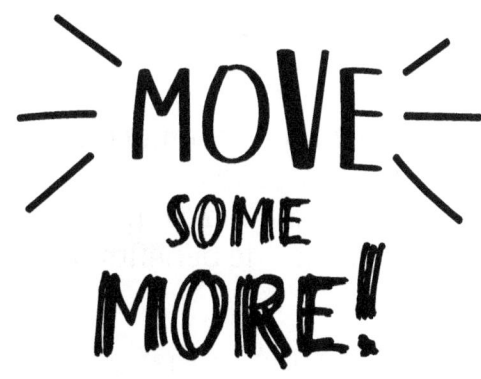

Solo-sports for spirit + Body
GET MOVING

(or you can join with friends!)

Weight-lifing
Skydiving
Scuba diving
Clean your room
Clean your house
Organize your closet! (Wardrobe)
Paint your room - or some furniture
Kayaking

Surfing
Swimming
Walking
Jogging
Skiing
Taichi
Qigong

Read Rapaciously, Learn Lasciviously

Most objectives need constant nurturing, consuming time and energy that don't always end with the results you expected. So, make an effort to feed and exercise your mind and the benefits will remain with you forever.

Seek knowledge constantly that defines your soul, your passion and your chosen profession; and over time you will be the better for it.

The easiest thing to read about is that which you love, so whether you enjoy painting, football or fixing radios, read about it.

Engaging in the activity is great; but imagine how much more you would appreciate it if you knew its history, technique and social impact through books. And if that doesn't tickle your fancy, read biographies about people you admire or even read horror stories if you enjoy gore. Just read.

If you want to be well versed in culture, on worldly matters or score well in your coursework, read voraciously. Make a commitment to reading and you'll find yourself an expert - respected and sought after in your field one day.

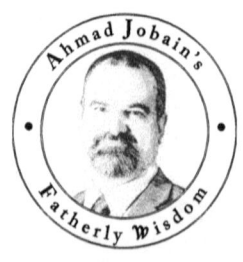

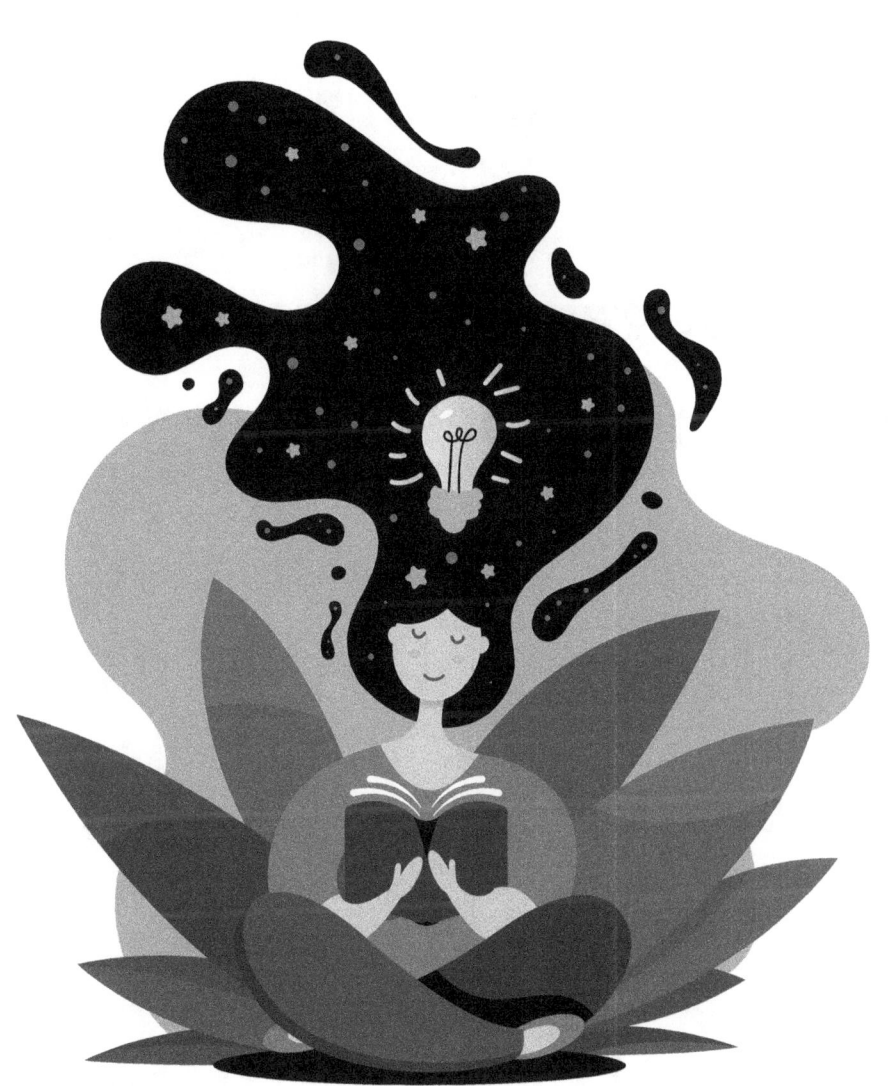

Nourish your mind and nurture your soul.

Be gentle on yourself when times are tough.

Remember you do have it in you to overcome, evolve + flourish (again)

DID YOU KNOW?

Experts agree
There is an increase in

STRESS LEVEL

for those who use

SOCIAL MEDIA!

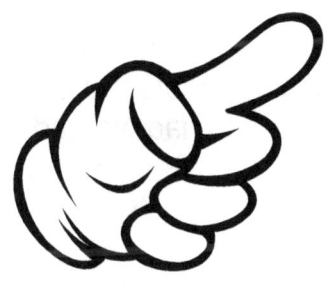

Tip:
Let others' posts 'roll off your back' + use the Golden Rule of "Do Unto Others as You Would Have Them Do Unto You" in YOUR posts & let's get closer to World Peace on social media!

Make a Plan & Accept the Consequences

When you hastily take on a task or consider only one approach – or when you multi-task out of a sense of rush, you increase the chances of a disappointing outcome. Whether on a tight deadline or a relaxed timescale, always practice scenario-planning and anticipate the outcomes - written down ideally; but at least considered mentally. Think about the context and facts that impact your mission and not only the result you expect.

Here are some things to keep in mind

1) bigger is not always better;

2) assumption without inquiry may lead to error, so gather as much information as possible before taking action;

3) always consider what the simplest solution is rather than what would be the most impressive (and then decide which to pursue!);

4) don't make a hasty decision;

5) once you've made a choice and taken action, accept the outcomes without beating yourself up if something doesn't turn out the way you had wanted. And, plan better next time!

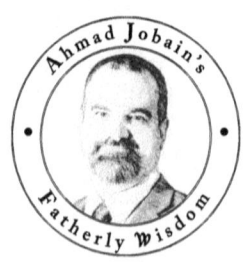

Live Aloha

Consider that.

International much?

QUICK! In 60 seconds, name 10 nations that **do NOT** contain the Letter "A". Okay, take another 5 minutes.

_____

_____

_____

_____

_____

_____

_____

Avoid Perfection

While you absolutely must become an expert in whatever profession or hobby you decide to pursue (through reading, training and practice), never believe that you must get every, single, little, detail just right before you start taking on projects or tasks. Just do the best you can within the deadline you've got.

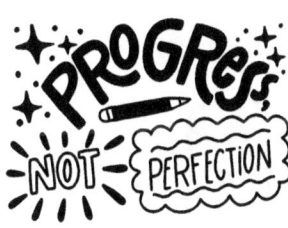

I learned this valuable lesson while preparing for the marketing of real estate projects in a highly competitive environment. I stressed over getting the right engineering designs, consultant fact sheets and other details before launching any project.

When I pushed for delaying a launch until I had all the right information, the company owner admonished me, stating that if we waited for all that, competitor properties would be sold instead of ours. He was right. There were several solutions I could have implemented to manage the shortfall in content without having to be a perfectionist.

So, while you should take precautions and consider conditions, you must move forward even when circumstances are less than ideal, otherwise you may miss out on opportunities far more beneficial than those that may come after the precision you sought.

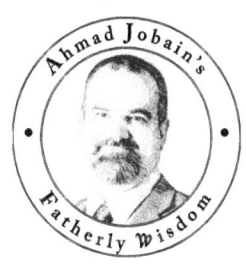

Recycle!
Upcycle!

Bring more biodegradable into your life.

Start Saving! Staple a perfectly good piece of monetary currency here

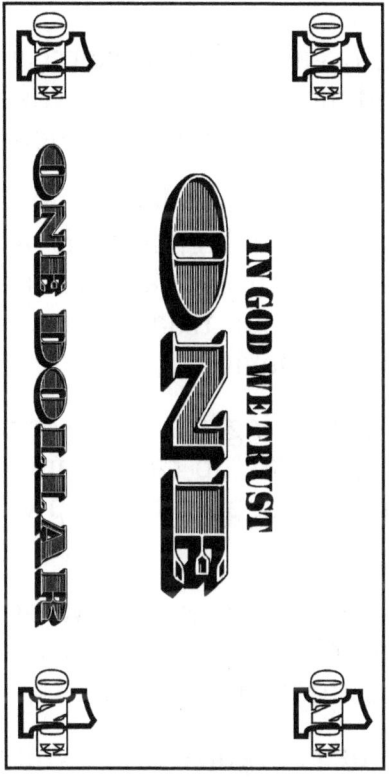

You may need it if the quarantines continue longer.

Make your Place & Be Seen and Heard

This means two things: be disciplined and respect order, for yourself and others. Make sure you neither take someone else's turn nor allow others to usurp yours, as long as you have the power to nonviolently do so.

Be structured, organized and exercise self-control at all times; and most importantly when interacting with people whose actions may influence your fate.

Being anything else may lead you to reckless, irrational decision-making; and as a result, can give others permission to take you for granted or misdirect a conversation from their wrongdoing to your emotional behavior.

Whether you're standing in a queue or participating in a work group, speak up calmly and deliberately if you're being browbeaten or simply stand tall if you're not.

In the movies, people who excel at what they do and overcome great obstacles eventually enjoy praise, recognition and material rewards.

If you want to be recognized, you will need to put yourself forward. Subtly sing your own praises by promoting achievements you've made as part of a team.

Submit your work to awards competitions and reach out to the media for coverage.

Create a binder or scrapbook to keep track of your successes and use this as a portfolio of your efforts and results (this will come in handy in the future!)

Shyness or pride may prevent you from putting yourself forward; but know that these sensibilities are self-destructive. If you don't speak for yourself no one else will be your voice.

You need not see yourself as vain by highlighting your accomplishments – just consider that the alternative is inviting obscurity, regardless of how good you may be.

By hoping others will act in your interests because you think you're a hard worker, you hand control of your image, and often your professional growth, to those who are preoccupied with their own agenda.

So, make sure you are visible even when others don't present you the opportunity to be. Just do it with class. Not many like a self-promoter.

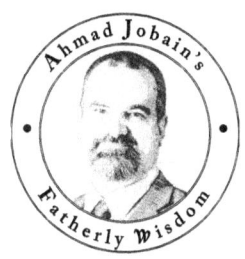

Be your own best Advocate!

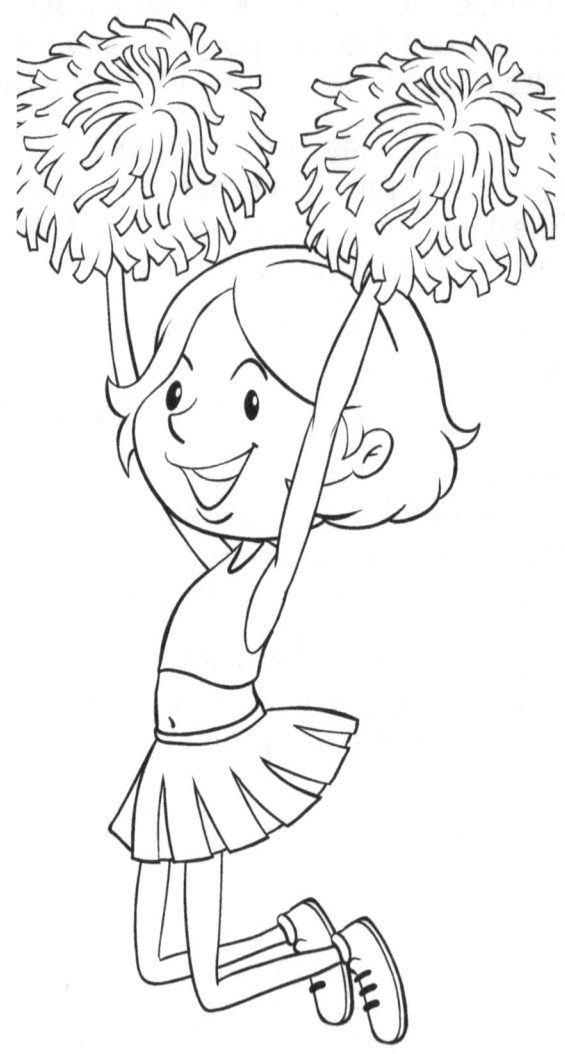

Cheerlead for You!

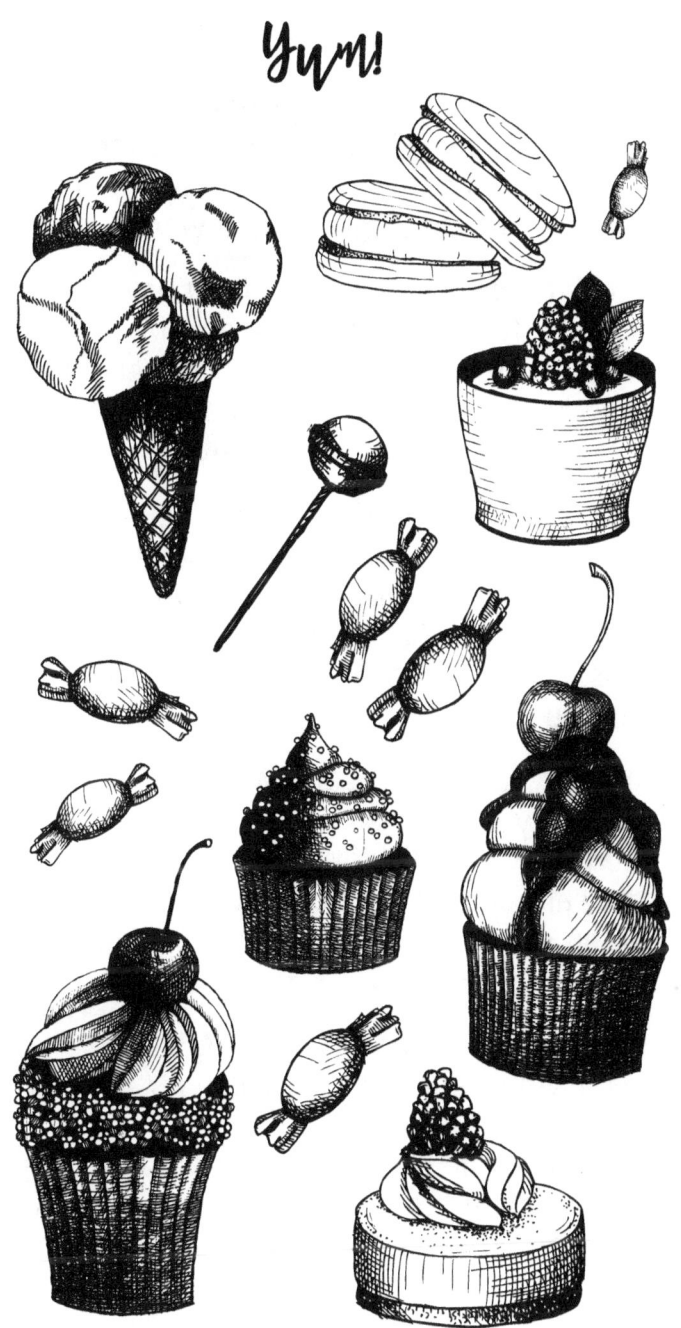

Minority Rules & Identity

If you are a minority (whether non-white living in a white majority or white living in a non-white majority) sometimes you may find there are elements of the majority that are discriminatory toward you.

Every society has those within it that have a neurotic obsession with The Other. These are the people that may have an inferiority complex or in their ignorance they may judge based on differences and this often starts with skin color, unfortunately.

And, the rise of bigoted nationalism is not going to disappear and hence you may be in the unenviable position of having to prove you're a decent, worthy part of society. Do that by managing your emotional reactions, knowing the laws and being the smartest at what you do.

You may be called derogatory names (I hope not) or feel uneasy in the way people look at you or talk down to you. Know that if these situations come your way, they are not a reflection of who you are; but of the person or group through whom your patience is being tested.

Just be the best ambassador you can be for your beliefs and origins; and be the best at what you do as a profession to help minimize the absurdity of prejudice. Pretty soon, you may find you win them over.

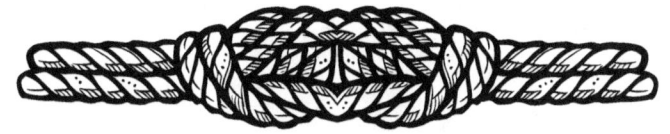

"When you reach the end of your rope, tie a knot and hang on"

ABRAHAM LINCOLN

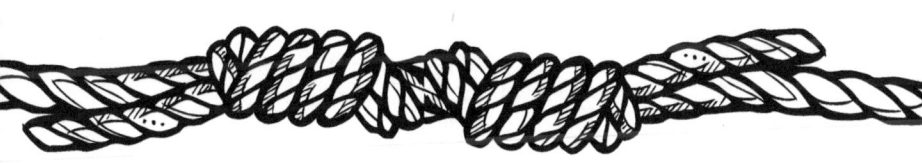

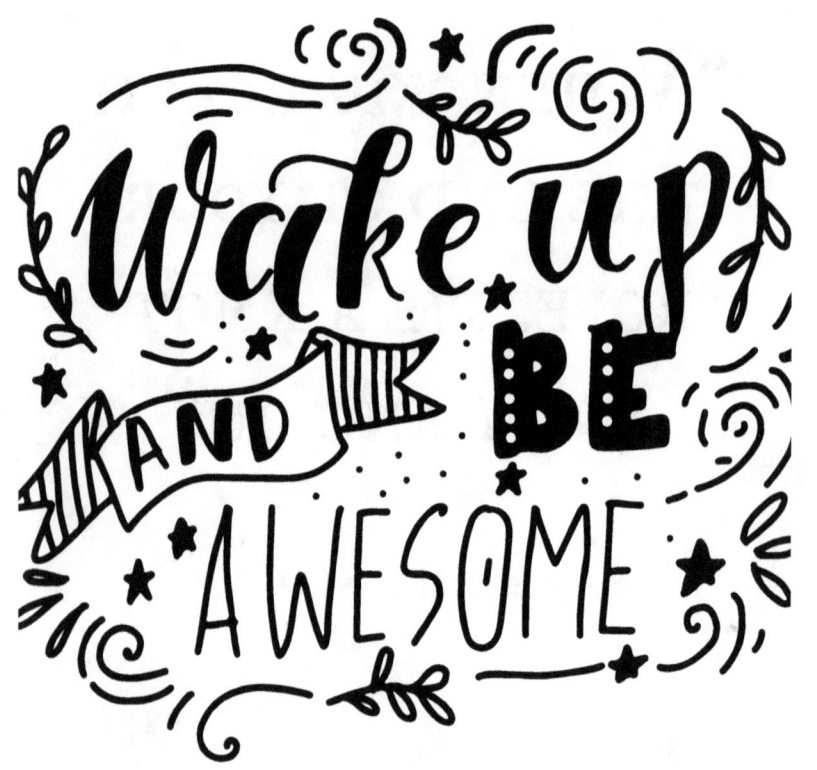

Dare to Be Different

Change is difficult. Most individuals stick to the comfort-zone of social norms and most external environments demand conformity.

The familiar feels safe and is easier to manage. You must disrupt the routines to which others are accustomed if you want to make your mark.

Of course, it isn't enough just to be the odd one out. You must match it with skills or provide a solution to problems people have.

So, if all factors are equal and you are as good as the next golfer, surgeon, singer or teacher – whatever you decide to be – make sure you are different in a way unique to you. It could be your clothing style, haircut, or just something you do, like a sport.

"People remember a standout."
Dad

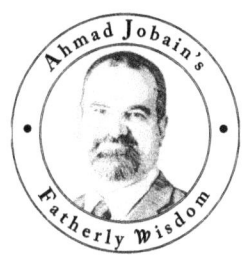

DOODLE
your cares away here

It's only TEMPORARY

(**NOTHING** - for better or worse, stays the same, **CHANGE** is the only constant)

If you feel:
Lonely, discouraged, upset, angry, confused, uncertain

1. Keep your head high

2. Keep the faith

3. Believe that better times are ahead.

"Just one small positive thought in the morning can change your whole day"

...and that's important to maximize the day because...

"There are only TWO days in the year that nothing can be done. One is called Yesterday, one is called Tomorrow.

TODAY is the RIGHT day to LOVE, BELIEVE, DO and mostly LIVE."

Dalai Lama

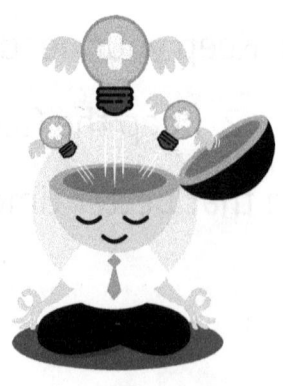

Life Isn't Always Fair

Although we want to believe justice will always prevail, unfortunately that's not always the case.

Growing up, you likely whined about the lack of equal treatment among you and your siblings or how some teachers treated you. You joined the 59% of Brits and 46% of Americans who believe life isn't fair, according to a 2017 YouGov survey.

The fact is, you're probably right half the time; and wallowing in self-pity the other half.

Hoping for fairness is giving yourself permission to complain, blame your lack of progress on circumstance and/or the absence of luck on 'the unfairness of it all' and someone else having dealt you a raw deal.

Having a positive outlook, skill or talent will help you succeed; but only determination despite inequity will make you a success.

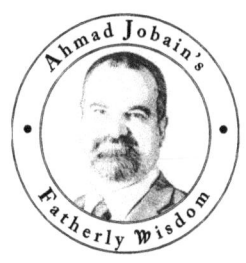

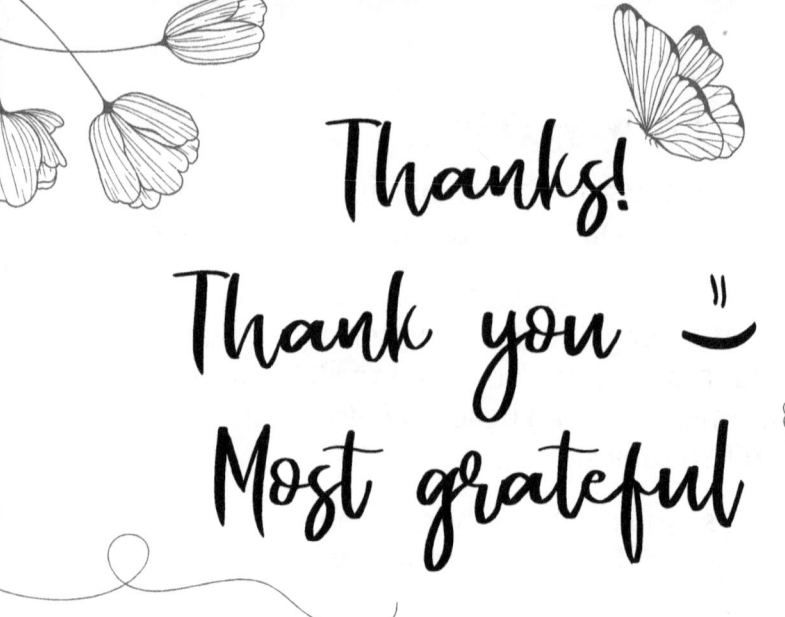

Thanks!
Thank you 😊
Most grateful

Make a list of those you should share these sentiments with, then...Do it!

Who	Why
1. _____	_____
2. _____	_____
3. _____	_____
4. _____	_____
5. _____	_____
6. _____	_____
7. _____	_____

What are you thinking about right now?

Your Body Speaks Volumes

There's a reason I tell my own kids to stand up straight, speak slowly and dress well. People perceive you as much by what they see as what you say.

The first person in the Western world to write down the effects of body language was Francis Bacon, a 15th century philosopher and politician, who addressed the matter with King James the First, noting: "For as your majesty sayeth most aptly and elegantly: 'As the tongue speaketh to the ear so the gesture speaketh to the eye.'"

Words spoken will be far better received from a well-groomed person dressed well and with good posture than by a slouch in tattered clothing uttering the same words.

Be conscious of what you look like, whether your breath reeks, how your eyes move and how straight you walk when in the presence of peers. Whether you like it or not, these details will affect how they treat and respond to you.

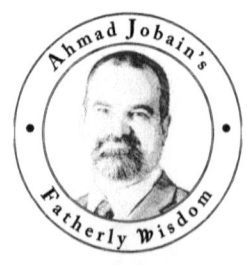

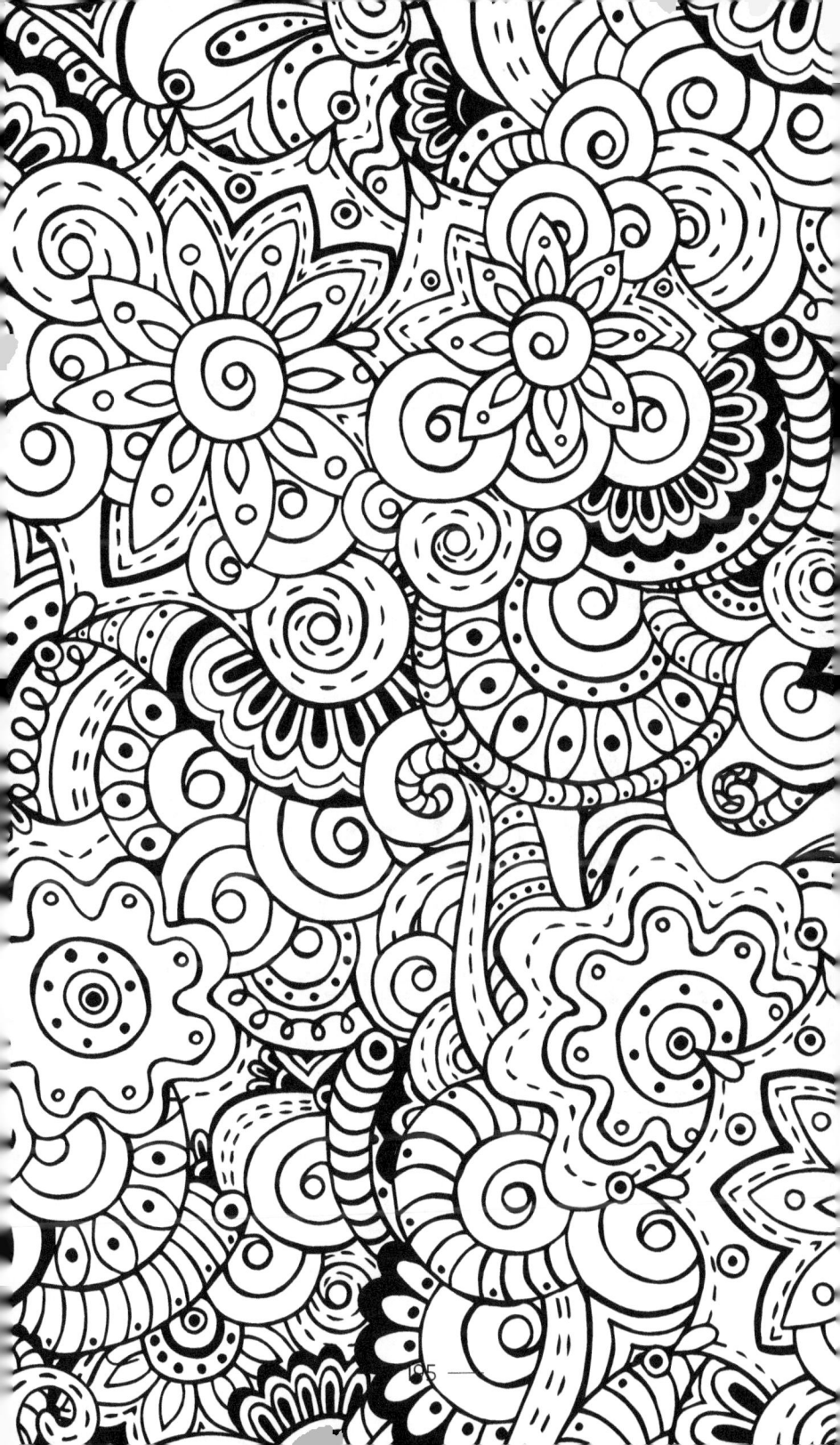

It's less stressful to live an honest life. Remember:

"A lie can travel half way around the world **while the truth is putting on its shoes.**"

Mark Twain who also said, **"If you tell the truth, you don't have to remember anything."**

See!

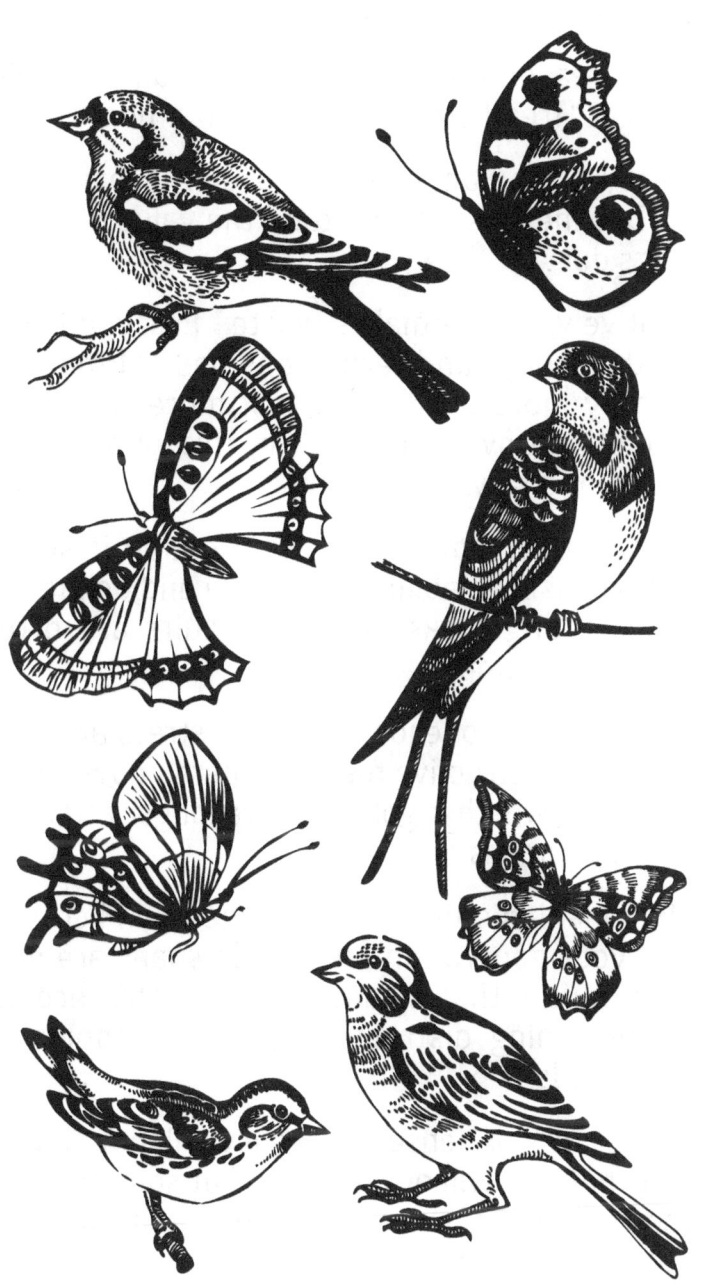

What's your Hurry?!

There's a reason my Arab ancestors came up with the adage: "Tread slowly, for I am in a hurry."

Sure, they didn't want to get run over by a marauding camel; but they also understood the value of giving a task its due.

Alternatively, "haste makes waste." Everybody's in a rush these days and technology has not made us necessarily more productive, just more connected and sometimes overwhelmed. Try this: unplug, take your time and slow down a bit.

In the quest for immediate gratification it seems many have lost the ability to be slow and deliberate when executing tasks and the results are often sloppy and incomplete.

Our impatience also leads to greater stress and self-defeating, or destructive feelings. There's now even a debate about whether goldfish have longer attention spans than humans.

A 2015 Canadian study commissioned by Microsoft showed your generation's attention spans are now eight seconds – that means it takes eight seconds before becoming distracted. Goldfish reportedly last 9 seconds!

Your eagerness or sense of urgency will not change the fact that you will only get good at something or get the best out of work you're doing, if you take time to carefully apply yourself to that thing.

Whether learning to play an instrument, building a robot, or going for the high score on Call of Duty, figure out the way it works, learn about it, practice it, then apply it; and take your sweet time doing so. Practice!

Recall: "Practice makes perfect", that's a generations old saying for a reason. And, when all else fails, remember the story of the Turtle and the Hare.

"Slow and steady wins the race." More often than not.

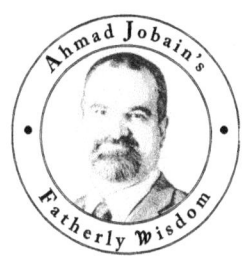

If you're
STRESSED OUT
about things that may seem are out of control like politics, environmental or social issues – or even closer to home with friends or family –

take a deep breath,

take a moment to consider the circumstances, positions, and rationale of the other side of the issues.

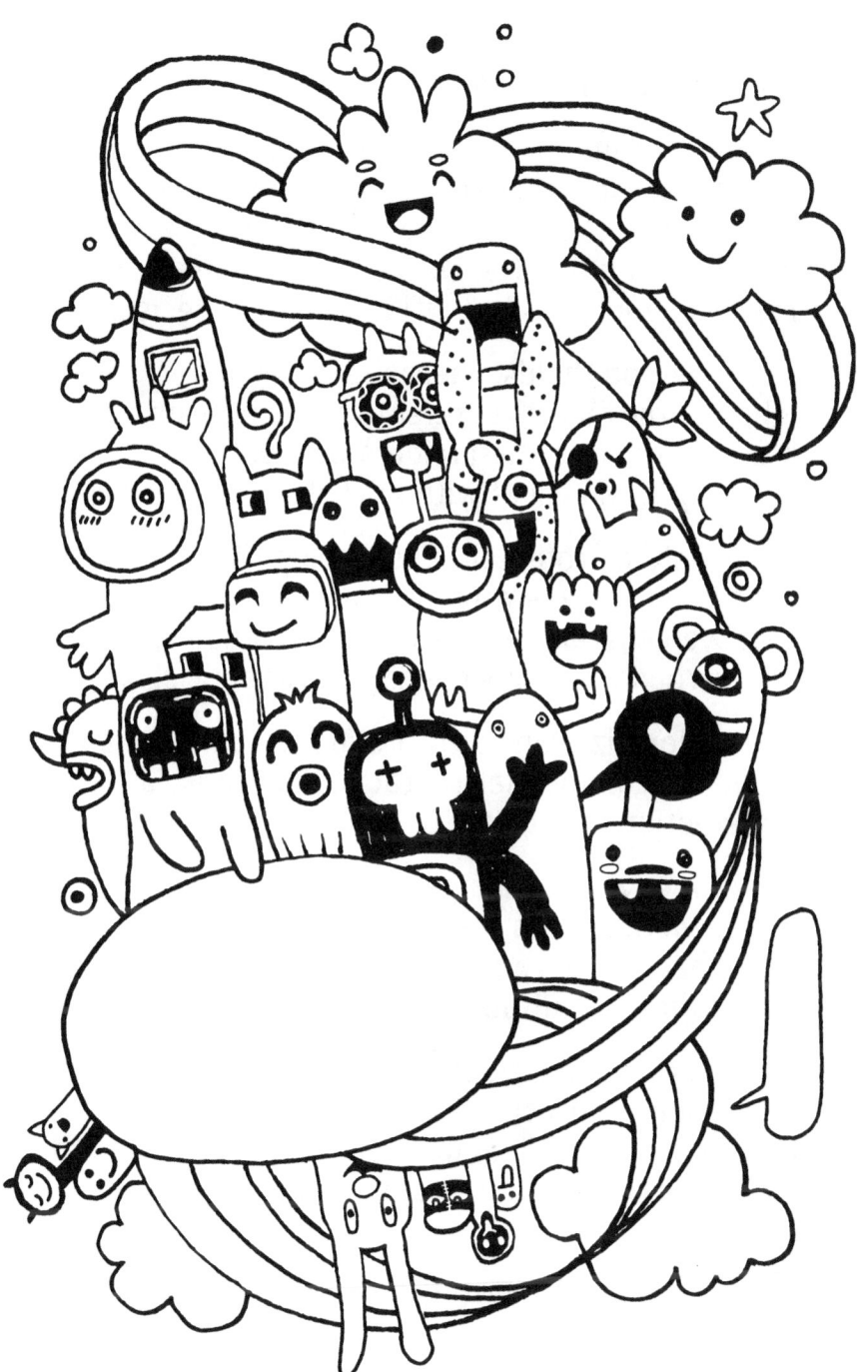

Listen, Think, Speak

In any argument, debate or dialogue, let others express what they want to say without interruption or correction. Learn to be the last to speak if you wish to command a conversation, earn people's respect, and possibly influence their decisions.

Each person holds their views relatively firmly, whether the facts they refer to are reliable or not; and it behooves you to first understand what they believe before you can agree with or challenge those beliefs.

Dan Ariely, a professor of psychology and behavioral economics, makes a point in *Predictably Irrational* that we generally reach conclusions then shape the truth around our convictions to give them legitimacy.

This rationalization has profound relevance to social as well as commercial interactions because it means our emotions are linked to our "truth."

If you try to change a perception without acknowledging its value to its holder, you will probably make your counterpart hold that view even more stubbornly.

Whether you are negotiating a salary, discussing a decision with your parent or significant other or hearing out a colleague, never prejudge. Let the other party feel you understand their views.

Know your value and the contributions or benefits you bring to the situation, declare your proposed offer, express your concerns and expectations.. This is nothing new, by the way; yet so few seem to communicate what they want and then are disappointed when they don't get what they had 'in (their own!) mind.'

We interrupt this page for a MOM-ism:

"I have such faith in you that you'll go far but first, listen and pay attention. **Concentrate**!"

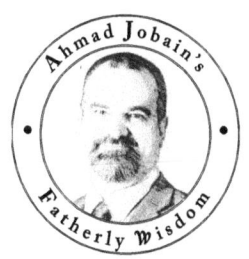

What is the first thing that comes to mind when you see this?

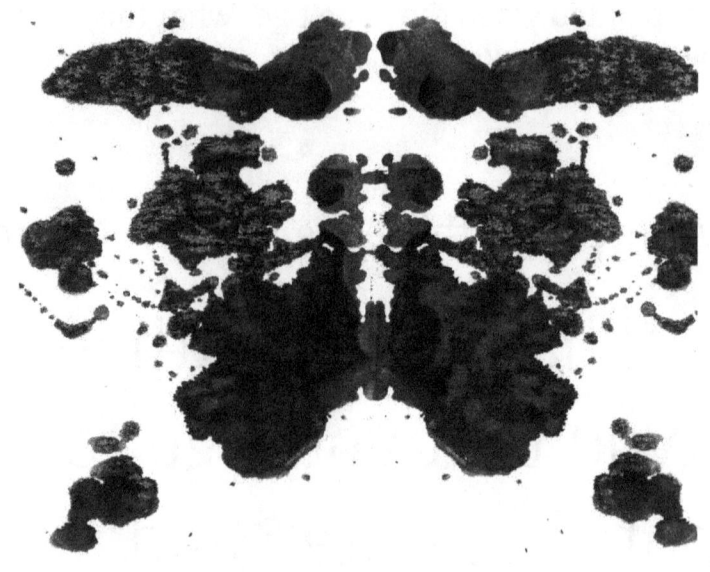

Disclaimer: you may need professional help. ask your mother.

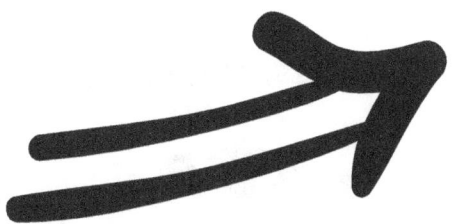

Pay it Forward

(When you're fortunate because of an act of kindness by another, you too then share the good juju + do something good for someone else

Keep some + Pass on the rest

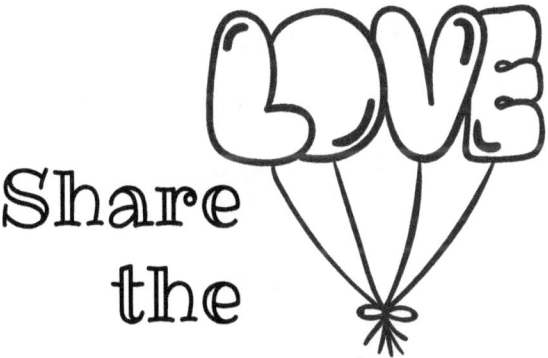

Share the LOVE

you can always spare a little of what you have with another who has less. And, sharing feels good too!

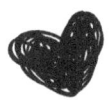

Decompress, Detach, Unplug

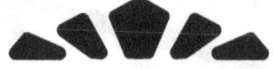

Switch off or silence your phone

Avoid checking social media feeds and status updates

Turn off your camera during video sessions for a bit

Try it a little bit each day until soon it becomes a healthy habit

Note: This is a tough habit to create. Take baby steps.

Humility is Overrated

No-one likes a conceited know-it-all; but most self-centered people rarely worry about how the powerless see them. They generally bulldoze their way through life, manipulating those in their path as it serves them through criticism, belittlement, self-righteousness or old-fashioned bullying.

You must temper your humility especially when dealing with conceit.

Excessive humbleness lets others get into your head, especially those who seek out perceived weaknesses to leverage. Eventually you will lose respect for yourself as others will if you don't keep your modesty in check.

Never let anyone believe they have power over you. The moment you sense someone being haughty, walk away to avoid wasting your time.

Always be true to yourself, confident in your mind that no person is better (or worse) than you.

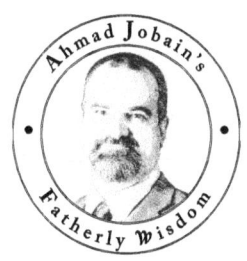

Release any negativity! Doodle Un-words to describe this pandemic.

Un-

Un-

Un-imaginable

Un-

Un-

Un-

Un-desirable

Un-

Un-

Un-

If Life gives you Lemons make Lemonade

Think of your BFFs and all of the

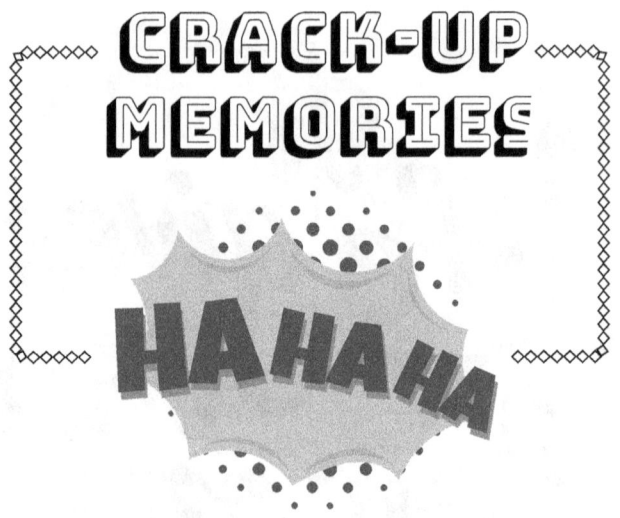

THEN SEND THEM A NOTE TO REMIND THEM

P.S. These are usually the friends you'll have forever

Peee.S.S. Have you ever laughed so hard you almost peed your pants?

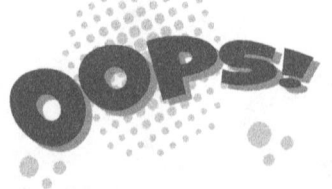

Tell that story!

Perspective & Perseverance, a Powerful Combo

Everything in life is a matter of perspective, so keep yours constructive.

Cultivate such traits to strengthen your character every chance you get. And, appreciate all you (already) have.

No matter what calamity you experience, it will rarely match Mark Tatum's. He contracted a fungus while gardening at his Kentucky home which resulted in the loss of his eyes, nose, cheeks, teeth and the upper roof of his mouth, earning him the moniker "the man without a face."

Despite this life-altering incident, he remained a proponent of perseverance and contentment; and he toured the country as a motivational speaker until his death in 2005.

Note from Mom:
"There is ALWAYS someone worse off than yourself" A powerful perspective to embrace and one that will keep you from feeling sorry for yourself. xo

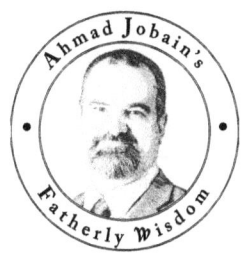

IN THE SCHEME OF YOUR ENTIRE LIFE, BEING HOMEBOUND A FEW MONTHS DOESN'T MEAN THAT MUCH

insh'allah, God willing, it's not the end of the world.

There has been a tragic surge of suicides in 2020.

PLEASE REACH OUT IF YOU ARE HAVING SUICIDAL THOUGHTS.
See next page for contact details.

We all struggle sometimes. KNOW THIS:

You are loved (by those you may not even know). We love you.

Suicide is a **permanent solution** to a **temporary problem.** You would leave a wound for many that would never heal.

IF YOU or someone you know is considering suicide, caring counselors are available 24/7. Confidential help in the US (even for non-Americans) can be found on the National Suicide Prevention Lifeline by phone at **1-800-273-8255** or by online chat at **suicidepreventionlifeline.org/chat/**.

A counselor will listen to you, understand how your problems are affecting you, provide support, and share resources that may be helpful.

If you are in USA and **feeling *deeply depressed***, or **worse**, ***having feelings of suicide***, or if you're in need of an anonymous, free ear to express you thoughts and feelings, reach out below. PLEASE, this is a personal request, PLEASE reach out if you are in need.

You are not alone and help is available

Youth & Teen Hotlines

National Youth Crisis Support:
1-800-448-4663

National Adolescent Suicide Helpline:
1-800-621-4000

Youth America Hotline:
1-877-YOUTHLINE (1-877-968-8454)

Covenant House Nine-Line (Teens):
1-800-999-9999

Boys Town National:
1-800-448-3000

Teen Helpline:
1-800-400-0900

TeenLine:
1-800-522-8336

Youth Crisis Support:
1-800-448-4663 **or** 1-800-422-0009

Take the online depression test at www.depression-test.net

Suicide Hotline

Suicide Hotline:
1-800-SUICIDE (2433)

Suicide & Depression Crisis Line:
1-800-999-9999

National Suicide Prevention Helpline:
1-800-273-TALK (8255)

NDMDA Depression Hotline – Support Group:
1-800-826-3632

Veterans:
1-877-VET2VET

Crisis Help Line – For Any Kind of Crisis:
1-800-233-4357

Additional Support

Panic Disorder Information and Support:
1-800-64-PANIC (1-800-647-2642)

Parental Stress Hotline:
1-800-632-8188

Help Finding a Therapist:
1-800-THERAPIST (1-800-843-7274)

Alcoholics Anonymous:
1 212-870-3400 www.aa.org

Drug Treatment & Hotline:
Substance Abuse & Mental Health Services Administration
1-800-662-HELP (4357)

Thanks to Dana Zarcone

Afterword

Realities & Reflections

As we headed into 2020, no-one thought that this was going to become one of the most challenging years for us all. When the news of a Coronavirus pandemic arrived, politicians in all countries tried to cope with the challenges posed by this new and uncertain situation – with varying levels of success it would turn out.

Although it was rapidly recognized that the virus was mostly a lethal disease of the elderly or others with preexisting conditions, measures were taken to curtail its effects by imposing drastic measures also impacting the young.

Under these auspices, the young were forbidden to see and hug their friends. Schools were closed, social distancing was mandated and large swaths of the economy were closed down. People were ordered to stay home and not see friends as well as extended family.

Daily news was disseminated about the horrors of the disease and how the healthcare system was being overwhelmed. Supply chain disruptions were obvious to all that took a trip to the grocery store to buy basic necessities.

Many lost their jobs and especially in parts of the world with very poor social safety nets, poverty became that much more prevalent and acute. This of course has deep ramifications on the way we perceive the world and brings about angst as we wonder what tomorrow will be made of.

Thinking about this as a war-like situation is not that far-fetched. This had deeply troubling psychological effects on young and old as it became obvious how frail the system we depend on for day to day life really is.

The collateral damage of this mandated change in behavior was not considered much in the early days. However, it is obvious as school closings linger and parents lose their livelihoods that the impact on mental health will be felt for much longer than the virus will persist.

For poor countries, the prospects to overcome poverty as been dampened that much more. The young can rightfully fear that they may not have the ability to get ahead as they may have been led to believe.

It thus comes as no surprise that many children under COVID 19 lockdowns have feelings of anxiety. For those having lived a carefree life with ample social contacts, a majority now struggle with boredom and feelings of isolation. Especially for the adults who are naturally distancing themselves from older/aging parents and see social interactions with their peers as the most important part of life, the sacrifices demanded by society are huge.

Being locked down with parents, especially in small apartments, in many cases was a sacrifice of epic proportions for adolescents and adults alike. Some situations were exacerbated by domestic violence, and in such cases the deleterious effects on one's psyche can't be overstated.

It's become both obvious and imperative that children must be provided greater social contact. Outdoor play, interfacing with friends and peers as well as opening of schools will help if implemented prudently with utmost precaution. Wherever possible, a psychological support system for the young must be put in place. The young have already sacrificed immensely and need to be taken care of properly.

In this book, you have read snippets of first-hand accounts of the meaning of the lockdown on young heroes of the year 2020 across the world.

Let their stories of ultimate resiliency be an inspiration to us all and let's all hope the path forward will be swift and positive for the many.

The famous second wave of infections is not an excuse to keep young children in limbo, expecting that the collateral damage is well worth the effort. There is a time of diminishing returns. Responsibly returning the life of the children to normalcy must be viewed as a top priority. Since this virus fortunately spares the vast majority of young people, it is hopeful that this can be accomplished.

Jose de Chastonay, Ph.D., Medical Microbiology and Bacteriology, Switzerland

Living, Learning and Embracing Change

- "Just when the caterpillar thought the world was over, it became a butterfly." – English Proverb

- "The trick is to enjoy life. Don't wish away your days, waiting for better ones ahead." – Marjorie Pay Hinckley, Author

- "Sometimes unforeseen opportunities emerge from the remnants of life's challenges. Sometimes it is possible to transform tough times into great growth and success." – Kay Douglas

- "Sometimes we have to lose something precious in order to gain something priceless." Author unknown

Acknowledgment

We hope that you've enjoyed this book and gained greater perspective on the bigger picture that is your life. After such a unique and trying time for many - anything that you take away that reaps positive impact renders this book a success as it's purpose was to provide uplift for a situation that's been a real downer.

Having been on sabbatical for a number of years I have been largely working and studying at my own pace and largely from the comfort of my home office. Over the course of the pandemic not much has changed for me – except that I created a wide-scale global initiative, the SDGs Challenge, to encourage and engage global citizens to unite to help solve the world's most nagging troubles – those defined by of the UN as the 17 Sustainable Development Goals (SDGs).

The cornerstone of this book is derived from 18 young team members, many whose teams created winning Solutions for the SDGs Challenge. These truly dynamic youngsters should be an inspiration to us all – they were for me and it's with much love and awe I thank them for the gifts of uplift that they've shared herein.

Special thanks to those who were instrumental in introducing contributors for this book – the indefatigable Linda Staheli, founder of the Global Co-Lab Network's SDGs Hubs and Lisa Martin and members of MUN Impact, especially Grace Makazawa of Lesotho for her facilitation skills and unending enthusiasm.

This book would not have been possible without Dubai graphic design czar, Rabab AlHaddad, whose patience I tried at every turn. Much love and respect for her artistic talents, numerous contributions and work ethic.

Special appreciation to one of our Challenge benefactors and author of this book's Afterword, Switzerland's Jose de Chastonay, Ph.D., Medical Microbiology and Bacteriology.

Much gratitude to Ms. Viva Goettinger of USA for sharing her expertise in the field of therapy and authoring this book's Foreword. Viva's connecting of a scientific topic with the simplified concept of 'making lemonade' provides for the perfect jump off point and invitation for reflection — for young and old alike.

Immense appreciation for author Mr. Ahmad Jobain, who imparts his advice throughout as only a father could with his "Fatherly Wisdom" pep talks.

Last but certainly not least, thanks galore to the SDGs Challenge team lead by Ambassador Eric A. Robson, with graphic design support by Irénée Isingizwe and proofreading by our news desk editor, Andrew Abell.

The "Global Citizens Innovative Solutions SDGs Challenge" is a 10 year initiative that runs over a rolling 100 day period annually starting each year on Earth day. The program will sunset in 2030 as will the SDGs.

This year on April 22, teams came together, ideated, collaborated, created and planned tangible solutions to their chosen SDG. During the course of our pilot "Year 0" we gained participation from 53 nations – 85% from developing and emerging nations comprising 143 mixed teams (the great benefit of virtual participation) comprising 610 global citizens aged 4 to 65.

Join us for our 2021 SDGs Challenge installment.

#Resolve2Solve Earth's most vexing issues.

It's free, it's fun, and can fill your life with new friends across the globe.

Learn more at www.SDGsChallenge.org

Whatsapp us on +1 240 281 0307

About the Author

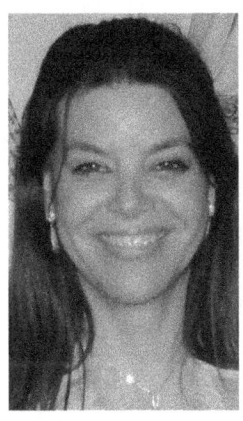

Lisa La Bonté is a technology investor, global emerging markets expert and business advisor who has designed and delivered programs of impact related to emotional intelligence, innovation, STEM, SDGs, and/or millennial workforce and economic development with foreign monarchies, The United Nations, US Department of State, NASA, and under Executive Order of the White House in cooperation with the US Department of Commerce.

Lisa holds and MBA in International Business, a Master of Science in Internet Strategy Mgmt. and is currently on sabbatical from her Dubai based youth development NGO while studying for a Masters in Journalism with a focus on International Security.

During the Covid-19 pandemic Lisa created the Global Citizens Innovative Solutions SDGs Challenge to cultivate greater involvement on the ground globally toward progress on the 17 UN Sustainable Development Goals. This book is an attempt to lift the spirits –or at least distract youth long enough for them to ride out the pandemic and return to their lives stronger, better motivated and more positive than ever.

You can follow Lisa on Twitter at **@UpliftingFYI** or visit **www.SDGsChallenge.org** and follow the SDGs Challenge: **@SDGsSolutions** on Facebook, Instagram, Twitter, LinkedIn and YouTube **#Resolve2Solve**